Sacred Coffee
A "Homesteader's" Paradigm

Also by Mark A. Zeiger:

Shy Ghosts Dancing: Dark Tales from Southeast Alaska

Read more from Mark A. Zeiger at AKZeigers.com/blog

Sacred Coffee
A "Homesteader's" Paradigm

Mark A. Zeiger

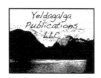

Yeldagalga Publications LLC, Haines Alaska

Sacred Coffee: A "Homesteader's" Paradigm

Published 2013 by Yeldagalga Publications LLC
PO Box 1316
Haines, AK 99827-1316
Yeldagalga.com
(907) 314-0242

ISBN: 978-1-61224-005-3

Printed in the United States of America

Cover and interior design by Mark A. Zeiger
Cover photo by Mark A. Zeiger

Another Fine Day from the album, *Busy Makin' Money* © 2007 Nancy Berland and Burl Sheldon.
Used with permission of the authors.
It's a great CD! Get yours today:
Send $17 to Burl Sheldon, PO Box 952, Haines, AK 99827
Also available at CDBaby.com and Amazon.com.

First Edition

Find more by this author at AKZeigers.com
This title is also available as an ebook.

TABLE OF CONTENTS

"And this, our life, exempt from public haunt,
Finds tongues in trees, books in the running brooks,
Sermons in stones, and good in everything."

—William Shakespeare, *As You Like It*

INTRODUCTION

Since 2006 my wife, Michelle, our daughter, Aly, and I have lived a sweet dream.

After years of pursuing a relatively simple, frugal life, we moved to a semi-remote, off-the-grid "homestead*," a small forest compound more than a mile from the nearest road, on the shore of Lynn Canal in the southeast region of our home state, Alaska.

Here, we have stripped away many of the trappings, urgencies, and concerns of modern western civilization to live closer to the land, working for ourselves to fulfill our own needs and wants.

In 2009 I began blogging about our lifestyle to let family and friends know how we fared. By publishing a blog we lessened the need to write similar versions of the same stories over and over. The Zeiger Homestead Website and Blog, at AKZeigers.com, has grown as strangers found it and began to read it regularly, drawing entertainment and inspiration from our adventures, misadventures, and musings. The blog expanded to offer specific advice on how to live as we do, recipes, and other

---

*One can no longer legally homestead in the traditional sense of claiming land and "proving it up" until ownership is granted by the government.

The term "homestead" is still used, but it refers to property on which the occupant lives off the land as independently as possible. When my family refers to our "homestead," that's our definition. We did not and could not have legally homesteaded this property. It's a homestead only in the sense that it provides us most of our living. This is why we try to remember to use the word homestead in quotes.

how-to segments. The blog has grown to nearly 1,000 posts on topics ranging from life altering to trivial, even silly. Newer readers have little chance of cutting to the pith of the blog, the core from which the best information can be gleaned. This book is an attempt to gather those posts in one convenient collection.

If you are not familiar with our Website, I urge you to log on now and take a look. Unlike this book, the Website features lots of photographs. Even though they barely do justice to the views we enjoy, and the sights we see living here, it might give you an inkling of why we love our home so passionately.

Visitors to the site often ask, "How can I live this way?" This book will hopefully answer that question for some. While it would be easy to say that you merely have to do as we did: fall ass-backward into the home of your dreams, it is at once far more complex than that, and far simpler.

In many ways, we lived this life long before we moved to the "homestead." Our parents were frugal, and we raised Aly the same way. Acquiring the property created the opportunity to focus our needs, wants, and desires, and to express them more fully. It also placed us in a position most people find unique enough to make what we have to say seem worth hearing. We didn't need the homestead to live a more centered, simple life, but our removal from "normal" American on-the-grid life helped immensely in that effort.

In an attempt, then, to answer that often-asked question, this collection of essays focuses on our paradigm—the philosophies and attitudes that underlie our lifestyle. It also includes some "how to," which explains various components of our operations. I originally wrote some of what follows explicitly to expound on the topic at hand. Others are included here because, even though they may not specifically address the topic, they help illustrate or otherwise illuminate it.

This book won't provide a blueprint for executing a plan to move off grid. We can only try to convey our own feelings, tell our own story, describe what happens to us, and explain how we view the world. Hopefully, our experience and opinions will help others create their own adventure.

We have not yet wholly realized our paradigm. Michelle currently works at a part-time job in town; I run a small publishing and Web design company, Yeldagalga Publications, LLC (Yeldagalga.com) from the homestead. We still purchase many of our necessities, and a good deal of non-necessities. We don't feed ourselves completely from our garden, from foraging, or fishing and hunting.

Even so, we are on the path, and whatever shortcomings one may choose to focus on, we live a life that we find in many ways far superior to the suburban lifestyle we left behind.

That is the essence of our decision to live the way we do: *to live a better life*. We're not trying to cut ourselves off from society; we're not turning our backs on everyone else. We don't aspire to live a "pure" life, totally free from fossil fuels and other non-renewables. While we see disconcerting signs that the status quo may not last very much longer, we have no firm, specific conviction that The End—economic, ecological, spiritual or otherwise— is inevitably near. If it is, we will be better positioned to deal with it than most, as we have largely shifted to the paradigm such an upheaval would require. But, our main impetus is to live more fully, focusing on enjoying our brief time together as a family, and pursuing the adventure of a lifetime in the process.

In this book I've collected some of my key writings on the subject of simple, centered, "deliberate" living. They encompass attitude, simple living, attuning to nature, frugality, family life, and on a more practical note, resource use. While I've roughly categorized each essay under one of these topics, most address all of the categories, explicitly or implicitly, in some way.

These are the most common themes of the blog; as it continues, we will no doubt write many more posts on these same subjects. The ones included here have already encouraged others who aspire to this kind of lifestyle. If you would like to read more on any topic, go to our blog and use our search feature. You'll also find that the original versions of these essays, in blog form, cross-link to other essays that are relevant to the topic being discussed.

Most of the following originated on our family blog. A few posts that more succinctly summarize our feelings on certain subjects come from a Website I used to collaborate with, Self-Reliance-Works.com. All have been revised from the original post; a few are unique to this publication. Hopefully, they will inspire you to pursue a simpler, purer, and perhaps more fulfilling way of life, as we have done.

A Disclaimer

The post that follows provides what may be our best disclaimer, pointing out the limits of our effort, its tameness relative to the everyday lives of many Alaskans, and our acknowledgement that we are not, in fact, "all that."

We're Not Alone:
"Roughing It" Within a Community

Because it's our blog, we get to focus a lot on ourselves in the posts. We also emphasize the rugged individuality of our situation.

However, we need to stress periodically that we're not alone out here.

We're a part of an off-the-grid neighborhood. If we're different at all, it's simply that we're a bit farther separated from the majority of homes over on the bay. Our nearest full time neighbors are as close as a quarter mile away.

We allude to the neighbors periodically. I don't say a lot about them most of the time, simply because it's none of our business to tell the wider world about them, or what they're doing. We're brave (perhaps naïve, even foolish) enough to broadcast our thoughts and activities to the world. That doesn't mean we have any right to expose our neighborhood in the same way.

Having said that, it's important to note that our neighbors have done much of what we're doing longer and better. They have patiently taught us, through explicit lessons and by example, much of what we've learned here. Some of it we doggedly learn in our own way. Doubtless our more experienced neighbors could improve on those tasks, methods, or practices. In addition, we owe an unrepayable debt to the previous owners of this property, who built the compound and set the "homestead" in place. All of our success rests squarely on their shoulders.

We ourselves seem to have very little of value to offer this community. That's long been a concern of ours, something we're seeking to overcome. We do what we can, and hope that it's enough, and taken in the right spirit.

It's also important to remember that in a wider sense, what we're doing here isn't unique. Other neighborhoods in our region are far more remote. There are thousands of Alaskans whose lives make us look like pampered city slickers.

We appreciate your willingness to read our blog, but if you want to learn how it's *really* done, I strongly recommend Seth Kantner's *Shopping for Porcupine: A Life in Arctic Alaska*. After that, you'll laugh at us for being so proud of our pathetic efforts a few miles from a town of any size. If you'd prefer something a little less extreme, there are other books and films out there that show truly off the grid, wilderness experiences.

What's my point? I don't want anyone to think that we're too full of ourselves. This is a humble effort, one that challenges our resourcefulness and capability, but it isn't anything earthshaking. We never undertook the blog to give that impression. Rather, it started as an easy way to let friends and family know what we're up to, and it's grown from there.

If at any time we seem to be taking ourselves too seriously, please use the comments section to bring us back down a notch or two. We'll certainly be better for it.

Originally posted on The Zeiger Family Homestead Blog November 30, 2009.

Attitude

There's little doubt that, had we been raised differently, or lacked adequate courage, initiative, or will, we never would have sought out our homestead lifestyle, nor would we have been able to maintain it. We've drawn inspiration from many sources to develop and sustain the right reasons and attitude for pursuing our lifestyle.

Living On the Edge: Security Through Insecurity

When the news came last autumn that the government had taken over Fannie Mae and Freddie Mac, our decision to chuck the standard suburban lifestyle, to head for the woods and off-grid—to live on the edge, in other words—made more sense than ever.

When we moved from Juneau, one of Alaska's larger towns (a truly relative term) to come to live on our "homestead" just over three years ago, we had a notion that something like this might happen. With relatives in the computer industry, we'd heard long before the year 2000 about the potential problems of Y2K. We realized that we in the United States are totally unprepared for the unexpected, whether that be a technology malfunction, like the narrowly-avoided Y2K scenario, an unthinkable event such as the World Trade Center collapse, a severe economic downturn like the current one, or a natural catastrophe: a hurricane, fire, or earthquake. We all like to think that things will be okay, that whatever comes, our elected and appointed officials will handle it for us. And, when catastrophes like Y2K are averted through incredible effort and expense, the public dismisses it as a hyped event that never presented a true threat at all!

Such "wisdom" allows us to go blindly back to our usual routines, confident that the next "chicken-little scenario" will be just as anticlimactic. Our family at least recognizes the potential such events have to disrupt society, and do not intend to trust that someone else will fix it for us.

Not that we made the move because of this...at least not entirely. The homestead fulfills our childhood dreams. As a bonus, it improves our family's situation should problems arise. We had far less access to good gardening, firewood, hunting, or fishing in our little Juneau suburb than we do here.

We quit our jobs and moved to our "homestead" to try our hands at living on the edge. We wanted to live closer to the land, growing or gathering what produce we can, hunting and fishing for the majority of our meat, maybe raising a few chickens now and then.

We are not completely independent by any means. Much of our food will always come from a store—after all, we can't grow our own coffee or black tea. We still have to pay taxes; we can't make most of our necessities as cheaply as they can be purchased elsewhere. We have a few monthly bills, insurance, Internet and the like. Even so, our need for cash has been greatly reduced by these new circumstances. We earn a little from various micro incomes, and I design Web pages using our satellite Internet connection.

There's a fair amount of risk involved with this lifestyle. The local fire department can't and won't come to our rescue should the cabin burn. Catastrophic illness would be just that. If we get injured, it's a long hike out for help.

On the other hand, stress is largely removed from our lives. As long as we focus on what we have rather than worrying about what we don't have, we are healthier. When we eat natural, unprocessed, homegrown foods, we are healthier. When we work and play as a family, and when those two concepts are intermingled, we are healthier. As we spend our days in activity and physical exertion, we are healthier. Also, good-hearted, educated, knowledgeable people surround us. Our neighborhood is comprised of people we trust.

As for the life of the mind, this has been a self-educator's dream! In the last three years we've learned more about electricity, fishing, hunting, gardening, water management, and myriad other topics than in the rest of our years combined. The learning curve is a steep one; class is always in session, and no one sleeps through the period or watches the clock! We are, in Thoreau's words, "living deliberately."

So, while wars rage and the economy tumbles, we are—all of us—living on the edge. Some of us, a little closer to it, may just have a better foothold.

Originally posted on The Zeiger Family Homestead Blog September 18, 2009.

Words To Live By

A daily feature of my Franklin-Covey Planner is an "inspirational" quote. I say "inspirational" because the Franklin-Covey people favor a few sources with which I vehemently disagree—inspiring, perhaps, but not to higher minded thoughts or actions. I also notice that since Mr. Covey bought the company, even adding his name to that of Benjamin Franklin, the revered originator of the concept on which the system is based, they try to "inspire" with far more quotes from Mr. Covey than from Dr. Franklin.

Most days, though, the thought is a worthy one. Occasionally, one really speaks to me.

Recently, I read this quote:

"The amount of satisfaction you get from life depends largely on your own ingenuity, self-sufficiency, and resourcefulness. People who wait around for life to supply their satisfaction usually find boredom instead."

—William Menninger

If you forced me to explain in a nutshell why we live the way we do on the homestead, this quote would cover it. When we made the decision to break from mainstream American life, we couched our arguments in much these same terms. Time weighed particularly heavily on me, as I followed a relatively clear career track at the time, working in a job that provided good pay, a level of security, union, benefits, retirement, and room for advancement. All I had to do was continue working until I reached my mid-60s, then retire in modest style.

Retire to what, though?

Would I have more time to spend with my daughter? She'll be in her thirties then, with a family and life of her own.

Retire to the homestead? I already wonder, most days, how much better this life might have been had we started it when we were 10 years younger. Starting it 10 years later would not work.

So, what? Take up *golf?*

"Living the American Dream," toiling as a good employee till I reach my late middle years would, indeed, be Mr. Menninger's "wait[ing] around for life to supply...satisfaction."

Maybe I'm too impatient. Or, maybe life's simply too precious to wait around for it to begin. Either way, these days I'm pretty satisfied!

Originally posted on The Zeiger Family Homestead Blog February 18, 2010.

Swimming Vs. Drowning

A while back, a fellow blogger used us as an example of living on reduced resources. He compared us favorably to another friend who also had no job, but who viewed that condition very differently.

He asked me if he could use us as an example. I introduced the prospect to Michelle and Aly, and as we mulled it over I was struck by one of the peculiarities of Alaskan life that bore a strong resemblance to the comparison the blogger intended to make.

I grew up swimming in the ocean in Southeast Alaska. When possible, we chose the warmest days and proper tides—as the tide rises on a rocky beach, the sun-warmed stones reduce the chill of the water slightly. Even when those conditions didn't exist, we sometimes went swimming anyway.

The life expectancy for a "man overboard" in our region, where the summertime water temperatures rarely get higher than the 40s, is about 15 minutes at best. How then can we swim in those same waters, sometimes for more than an hour at a stretch?

The answer, I believe, is positive mental attitude and intention. Deciding to swim, preparing for and executing that decision bear almost no relation whatsoever to accidentally falling into those same waters. If you had taken me from the beach, dried me, dressed me, took me out on a boat off that same beach, and shoved me in unexpectedly, I probably wouldn't have beat any endurance records.

My point is that I wonder if I can really be compared to my fellow blogger's friend? We took the plunge (if you'll forgive me) voluntarily, determinedly, even enthusiastically. This did not happen to us while we were making other plans—it *was* the plan! The blogger's unfortunate friend certainly didn't plan to lose his job.

It's all about positive mental attitude, and intention. You see it among firewalkers—they're out there calmly, coolly doing the impossible. To some, we're right out there with them.

It humbles me, gives me pause. I doubt it'll tempt me to try fire walking, though.

On the other hand, I have been laid off in the past, and we managed the situation quite well.

Michelle and I delayed buying a house or starting a family for the first 10 years of our marriage. I had chosen an exciting career path that provided no stability. Neither of the two intertwined goals could be pursued safely until I found a position that seemed secure enough to take these life-changing steps. Eventually, I found a job with a stable company in a town (Juneau) in which we could envision living for the rest of our lives. I quickly rose to a top position. We hunted for a house, and we started our family.

In August of the next year, we moved into our new house within a week of our daughter, Aly's birth.

In November, I faced the unpleasant task of telling Michelle that I had been laid off.

Of course we were scared. Of course we discussed our options long and hard. We made some rash decisions, muddled through, compromised, rationalized, and doubted. I won't go into the details, except to say that I spent the next six months as a "house husband" while Michelle's work supported us. I applied for jobs, tried moneymaking schemes that didn't amount to much, but mostly I cared for our infant daughter. In retrospect, those were the most precious six months of my life. I might have been more productive doing something else, but no job could have been more important!

Our frugal nature and practices saved us. We paid our bills, met our obligations, and ate healthily. Eventually, I found a job using skills I'd developed in parallel with my former career. Soon, I found a better job that paid more than my best paying position in my former field. Each new job brought increased pay, even though they often required me to learn new skill sets.

Now, sitting snug in the woods, getting by on subsistence, micro incomes, and savings, I sometimes lose sight of what I've achieved in the past. I forget that I'm not avoiding the "rat race" because I couldn't handle it, but because I've found a better way.

Originally posted on The Zeiger Family Homestead Blog July 9 and 11, 2010.

The Cost of Living

Recently, a reader commented:

"Ever since I can remember I have wanted [your] lifestyle. It's tough [where I live] because everything is about money. You are expected to work all year round for someone else and to not have any time to save food for yourself or make Christmas presents. I've always thought about Alaska as a possibility and I'm not afraid to work hard at an honest life. How can I do this? What did something like this cost you?"

Rather than replying to her comment directly, I realized my answer would be long enough for a post on the subject.

The first question: "how can I do this?" varies greatly according to circumstance, opportunity, and resources. In her book, *Made from Scratch: Discovering the Pleasures of a Handmade Life* (reviewed on the blog) Jenna Woginrich shows how to pursue a simpler, more self-sufficient lifestyle wherever one may be. She shows that location doesn't matter so much as one's desire to live the lifestyle. I heartily recommend this book to anyone who seeks a life like ours.

On the other hand, I'm not the best one to advise people on starting such a life. We're succeeding at it largely because we've generally been more frugal than most, willing to live a simpler lifestyle than most, and acquired many of the skills we need to live this way early in life. If that's not true for you, you may have a harder time adapting to the lifestyle.

As for cost, my initial response is that it cost us very little. That's because I thought first in monetary terms. We had earned and saved enough over the years to buy a home and eventually invest in a little bit of remote property. By the time we sold the house to pay for the "homestead," we'd built up enough equity to pay off the new mortgage in a very short time. Sales of most of the remote property helped as well. Financially, moving to the homestead compared favorably to moving to a nicer home.

Tallying the real costs presents a somewhat different picture.

We've reduced the time we spend working for others; the reader's observations on the matter are very similar to our own.

Devoting so much time and effort to working for a wage rather than directly for the family rubbed me the wrong way, and led to the choices we made that helped us change our lives.

On the other hand, we've had to make do on far less income. We've also lost the security (or illusion of it) of health insurance. We've had to forego family visits to a large extent, and accept that those will become even less frequent as we age. Almost everything we do takes longer, requires more planning and effort, and involves overcoming obstacles unknown to most of our countrymen in this modern age.

These are trade-offs, but so far, they've been well worth it. These "costs" buy us a larger sense of contentment, wellbeing, and satisfaction than most people know, more family time, more freedom. All in all, I'd say it's been well worth it, and I think most of the posts on this blog illustrate the myriad ways in which our lives are better—richer—for having chosen this lifestyle.

It is, indeed, the cost of living, and we're willing to pay the cost as long as we're able to do so in order to live the way we do.

Originally posted on The Zeiger Family Homestead Blog October 18, 2012.

Courage

I have had far too many opportunities in these last few weeks to meditate on the meaning and qualities of courage.

This lifestyle requires courage on many different levels. From dealing with wild animals to navigating rough water in small boats to living without many of the security nets our society relies upon, the demands on one's nerve weigh heavily.

Any fear we feel seems intensified by the contrast between our peaceful, largely stress-free existence and the occasional crisis. The usual calm has made us a bit more sensitive to surprises than "normal" people might be; by the same token, a real problem seems far larger than it might if considered against more common background stress levels. And, while I may preach a good line when it comes to dealing with fear, I often find myself close to despair when dealing with homestead crises, especially when they involve the electrical system.

If I have one nemesis on this homestead, it's our wind generator. We rely heavily on it operating properly, and enjoy many benefits when it does. When it doesn't, a crisis develops, and whatever courage I can summon is called upon to manifest itself.

The worst part about repairing or maintaining the wind generator has to be that so much of this work occurs on the tower. I am not unduly afraid of heights. As long as my balance is centered and my footing firm, I will stand comfortably at the edge of a precipice and look down. Take away the secure stance, and all bets are off.

Even 20 feet off the ground, if I have to cling precariously to stay aloft, I begin to worry.

I've assembled some impressive safety equipment, and almost perfected my method for climbing the tower, even as we built a new, cantilevered tower that can easily be raised and lowered when necessary. The need to climb the tower remains, however, and as I get older, I find myself less able to face this task. Each time I climb the tower, I feel I can't do it. Each time, I do it anyway.

Each trip up the tower has its own affect on me. Sometimes, I feel almost at home clinging to the pole, 20 feet or so from the near side rocks, 30 feet from the jagged beach rocks on the other side. Other times, the fear numbs my mind and impairs my thinking. I never know what to expect, other than the worst—hoping for better, but braced to do as much as I can in the time allowed.

The difference has to be a combination of weather conditions and my physical condition. As I tire from the various strains, as the scrapes, thumb crushing, and fatigue mount, my ability to remain aloft diminishes. I've learned to control my breathing, to avoid distractions, shift the position of my feet often, and to take pain relief medicine as soon as I return to the ground. Mostly, I focus on my resolve to accomplish my goals quickly and efficiently, and get off the tower as soon as I can.

I assume the fear will only increase as I continue to age. I assume there will come a day when I can no longer do it. All I can do is strive to put that day off as long as possible.

Wise people have stated that courage isn't an absence of fear, but the ability to take action in spite of fear. I cling to that definition, as I continue to do what needs to be done around here, despite the fear.

Originally posted on The Zeiger Family Homestead Blog January 27, 2013.

Optimism and Self-Reliance:
Interchangeable by Definition

At the risk of stating the obvious, optimism is key to self-reliance. I believed this to be true before hearing my sister, a Doctor of Psychology, speak on optimism, but she taught me that the tie is closer than I had suspected.

Many terms we regularly use have slightly different meanings than what has become commonly accepted. Optimism is one of them.

In clinical terms, optimism doesn't mean naïvely assuming that everything will always be well. Rather, optimism is the ability to look at situations from a standpoint of empowerment—to understand that if we need to change a situation, we can often find ways to do so.

By this definition, optimism practically defines self-reliance. An optimistic outlook inevitably leads to self-reliance, to a greater or lesser extent. The more I heard of my sister's talk, the more I realized that the two terms are almost interchangeable.

I'd always considered myself a realist: not a pessimist, but not a "Polly Anna/Always Look on the Bright Side of Life" optimist, either. Now I see that according to the true definition, I, and others like me (that probably means you) am an optimist, because I believe I have the power to change most situations. In essence, optimists are proactive, pessimists are reactive.

So, you don't have to be cockeyed about it, as the old song puts it, but you may be surprised, as was I, to realize that you are, in fact, an optimist!

Currently unpublished.

Self-Discipline, The Key to Self Reliance

Self-discipline. This is a good term, which, I confess I haven't given a whole lot of thought until recently. It's a phrase we hear all the time. I've never considered it a quality I particularly possessed, but I'm beginning to reassess that.

As I blog, I'm noticing a strong common thread. Self-discipline is key to virtually every aspect of self-reliance. It's also directly responsible for my family's success on the homestead.

After all, what is the primary ingredient necessary to accomplish any of the following?

- Self-directed learning through "unschooling"
- Living within one's means
- Becoming and staying debt-free
- Gardening
- Hunting
- Fishing
- Gathering fuel to heat one's home
- Learning new skills
- Using a day planner to manage time
- Achievement—*of any kind*

The answer: self-discipline!

I'm rather quick to downplay or dismiss my own accomplishments. I enjoy writing in a self-deprecating style. Perhaps that has kept me from realizing just how much my family has accomplished, and the important role self-discipline has played in those accomplishments.

Perhaps I hadn't thought much about self-discipline because it seems so natural. Both Michelle's and my parents ingrained it in us deeply. Both families modeled frugality and responsibility. I went through a long period of acquisitiveness, but it was always tempered by frugality, and it faded as I matured.

Michelle and I eliminated most of our debt around 2000-2002, probably earlier. We paid off everything except our mortgage. "Everything" included a brand new vehicle and about 5 acres of remote property. Our obligations were never substantial; we hadn't carried any credit card debt for about 10 years, despite using the cards for almost every purchase (in order to accrue airline mileage). If we did carry a balance, it was extremely small.

Once those debts retired, we increased our savings and contributions to retirement funds, and began pouring extra money into the principal of our mortgage. We did this while maintaining a comfortable lifestyle that suited us, and building a wooden sailboat in our driveway!

This is why I often talk about "falling ass-backward" into our "homestead." By the time the opportunity arrived, setting and achieving the goal of purchasing and moving to the property seemed simple!

Without self-discipline, none of it would have happened, and we would not have been successful in our current lifestyle. We planned effectively, we looked for every available financial advantage, and we achieved it.

I should add that being good at self-discipline is not the same as being expert at it. I confess to poor self-discipline in many areas. Or, perhaps there's difference here between self-discipline and self-control. I'm not presenting myself as a paragon to which others should aspire, I just hope to point out that some of the things we do simply won't work for those who don't have a firm enough grounding in self-discipline.

Originally posted on The Zeiger Family Homestead Blog November 29, 2009.

Waiting for Perfection

"One of the most tragic things I know about human nature is that all of us tend to put off living. We are all dreaming of some magical rose garden over the horizon—instead of enjoying the roses that are blooming outside our windows today."

—Dale Carnegie

Ever since I was a kid, I've strived for perfection in many ways, mostly the wrong ones. I actually pulled a "D" in junior high shop class—a disaster for an otherwise straight-A student.

We were building step stools. I built mine well, but I got caught up in trying to put a finish on it. I worked on it as I would a piece of fine furniture, trying to give it a mirror-like surface. As a result, I never completed the project, and earned the lowest grade short of complete failure.

About a month after receiving that grade, I suddenly realized the awful truth: had I achieved the finish I desired, it would have been completely destroyed the very first time someone used the stool for its intended purpose!

Lesson learned.

A friend who helped build our sailboat, *Selkie,* encouraged our efforts by teaching us about perfection. He stressed the difference between Platonic perfection and Aristotelian perfection.

As he explained it, Plato believed in perfection as an absolute ideal—a state that could never be reached in the real world. Aristotle saw perfection as that which falls short of ideal, yet can be achieved. In short, Plato might work for years to build a mathematically and aesthetically perfect sailboat, while Aristotle would be happy with a prime boat builder's axiom: "If it looks right, it *is* right."

I'm not a big fan of the Classical philosophers. I feel that we would live in a far more enlightened world if western society had not canonized these deep thinking, yet ultimately deeply silly men. Even so, remembering their differing views of perfection have helped us accomplish far more in life than we would if I had held true to my desire to achieve ultimate perfection.

These lessons, which embody Mr. Carnegie's views above, have allowed us to create the life we live today. Had we held out for perfection, our first view of the homestead would have led us to pass on it. If we expected perfection of ourselves, we would have long since given up on our efforts here. We've done well, but there's much to be done—so much that should be done before the homestead is perfect.

The plain fact is, perfection will never come. That doesn't mean we won't continue to work toward it. It does mean that as we do so, we appreciate, even revel in what we have.

Many people follow this blog because they plan to live like we do someday. Start now! Don't wait for the perfect (Platonic) situation; make what you have perfect (Aristotelian) as soon as you can.

Originally posted on The Zeiger Family Homestead Blog February 5, 2012.

Why Versatility is Key for Homesteaders

Several years ago, I entered an article competition on this title. I created a laundry list of make-do, self-teaching, and improvisation, condensed into an imagined conversation with a visitor to the homestead.

I could never say anything like what I wrote below to anyone. I may think it, but it's not in my nature to say it, at least not this way!

Nevertheless, it's a decent overview of the kinds of skills we've had to acquire to make a life for ourselves here on the "homestead." It's updated to reflect improvements we've made since the article first appeared on line.

* * * *

If you were to ask me how versatile a homesteader must be, I'd invite you to come see for yourself. Hike across the tidal basin and over the ridge to my homestead, perched on the ocean's edge in southern Alaska.

Here we are. The previous owner built the cabin by hand. That's a James washer; we use it to wash clothes. It's purchased, but we modified it to make it safe to use.

That's not an open pit outhouse; we use a home-built composting toilet system.

The contraption over there is a pulk, a harness-pulled sled. I built it myself to haul firewood and supplies.

Come inside for coffee! It won't take long since we installed the propane stove. I'd never used one before. I had to learn how to hook up the tanks with the proper couplings. Before that, I was happy to use the wood stove. We've gotten pretty good at cooking on it.

You like the hearth? We built that ourselves when we installed the wood stove, choosing rocks from the beach and mortaring them with cement. Beside it is a wood-heated hot water tank. We used to have a larger one, but we couldn't patch it anymore, and had to tear it out and replace it with this one. I had to change the plumbing and re-sweat the fittings to the new equipment. We rebuilt the drains in the sinks and replaced the shower spigots at the same time.

Would you grab the coffee jar? It's under the sink. The hose under there is our fire protection; it's tied into the plumbing. You'll also notice fire extinguishers everywhere, and smoke alarms and carbon monoxide detectors in all the buildings. All three of us have practiced knocking down a fire with an extinguisher at the Fire Department. Can you imagine municipal fire fighters responding to a call on this side of the ridge? We're completely on our own in that case.

Same with injuries, unless we can hike or boat out. We've got some first aid training, but we intend to get certified in back country emergency response next time it's offered. It's one of the few trainings available anymore that teach much more than how to stabilize an injured person until 911 sends the ambulance. That's not going to happen here.

A guest broke her ankle two years ago. She had a green-stick fracture. We made a poultice out of plantain, that flattened plant you see in the yard. She had it checked when she got home. That's when they discovered the fracture! She told her doctor about the poultice, and he said it was the best thing we could have done for her. Now we keep two pairs of crutches on the property just in case.

Be careful of those jugs, that will be rosehip wine in a few months.

Do you like that counter? I built it out of plywood. We recently surfaced and finished the one across from it, too. The same with the firewood box.

The box in the corner is the battery bank. The batteries were in the outhouse at first. We moved them inside so they wouldn't freeze. I vented it to the outside, relocated the controller boxes, rewired everything. I tied in the new solar panel array at the same time. The cabin wiring is getting old and we need more outlets. I intend to rewire the whole place soon. I've already tied the stereo and the Citizens' Band radio into the DC line. That inverter handles the AC requirements, but I put in a few DC outlets for our rechargeable tools. They draw less power that way. Where did I learn to work with electricity? Books, manuals, trial and error...the same way we learned to do everything else around here.

Let me show you around outside. Here are our boats: I built the three sailboats. The rowboats, kayaks and canoe are factory-built, but I've patched each of them over the years.

The gill nets there I cobbled together from odds and ends. I've also taught myself to throw a cast net. Mostly, though, we use our fishing poles.

Those are our crab traps. The one on the left is original store-bought, the rest I modified myself. The State changed the escape hatch requirements after they were built, and I had to make changes to them to be legal again.

You can see the garden's pretty well laid out now; that's my wife's doing. We're piling on seaweed to build up the soil, which is pretty thin. That's the greenhouse. My wife made the water catchment system. It'll automatically shut off when that bucket gets full. Those beds hold lettuce, five different varieties. The little green plant underneath is really tasty, too. My wife makes pesto with it, or we use it in salads. Most people consider it a

weed, but it's got more nutrients than a lot of leafy
vegetables. The cold frames are over there, where they'll
get better sun this winter.

Over there's our primary wood lot, where we cut
standing dead trees to buck and split for firewood. That
got a lot easier after I learned to sharpen the axes
differently for specific uses. I've got the tools and a
manual for sharpening the two-person saw, I just have to
read about it, then give it a try.

That? It's a moose track. The permit hunt's coming
up, I'd better clean my rifle soon and practice at the firing
range. We're working on our archery skills to qualify for
bow hunting. The voles? We shoot them with blowguns.
Mostly, though, minks and weasels keep their numbers
down. The predators may become a problem if we raise
chickens next summer. First we need to see if we can
figure out a good way to keep the chickens fed without
hauling bags of commercial feed over that ridge.

No, that looks like bear scat, but it's moose. It looks
like that when they're on their summer browse; the
nuggets come from woodier browse. Fooled us too, until
we researched it. I don't see any bear scat today, or I
could show you the difference between them.

You're right, there are a lot of mushrooms here.
From where we're standing, I see three varieties that are
safe to eat, but only two of them actually taste good. That
one is deadly poison, though.

We just overhauled the wind generator you see on
the left. It wore out. We have four old units like that. We
chose the best parts from among them and made a new
one, then painted and reinstalled it. When the one on the
right burned out a few winters ago, I had to climb up
there to disconnect and remove it, lower it, and send it
off for repairs, then haul it back up, put it back in place,
and reconnect it. I made a homemade safety harness and
lashed my longest ladder to the tower pole. Since then we

built a cantilevered tower from scratch. The generator burned out again, but we fixed it ourselves this time.

That dish gives us satellite Internet. We use it to help home school our daughter, and I design Websites freelance. We don't need much, since we have so few expenses here.

We might want to step inside, there's a nasty squall coming. How do I know? See the cat's paws coming across the water there? Then you see the pattern in that cloud cover to the south? Around here, that means rain. In flat country, that system would miss us, but the weather funnels up the fjord here. See, now you can tell it's raining on the mountains across the way. It'll be here about the time we get back to the cabin. Looks like it won't last long. We'll have a comfortable hike back to your car in about an hour.

What's the key to living here? I'd say it comes down to this: living in a regular neighborhood, you can do a few things for yourself if you want, then find someone else to do the rest, either hire a professional, or rely on the government to take care of it. On a homestead, to a far greater extent you do it yourself, find help to work along side you, or do without.

It's a good life! All you have to do is stay versatile.

Originally posted on Helium.com November 23, 2008.

"The Big Question" Requires a Follow-Up Question

It has almost become customary for presidential candidates to ask voters The Big Question: "Are you better off now than you were four years ago?" The incumbent hopes and assumes you'll say yes; the challenger hopes and assumes you'll say no.

In the current election, the question has been raised once again, so, like most Americans, I'm assessing the state of my wellbeing over the last four years.

Since the current president took office, I started my own small business. I didn't seek any loans or grants to start the business. I started it using our own funds. An investor injected a small amount of capital—$500—but I didn't need that investment to get started. It was just a good opportunity for both of us at the time.

By the next year, I showed a net profit. Clients are fairly thin on the ground, since people are nervous about spending money, but I'm pretty happy with the work I've been hired to do, and the clients seem to be as well. I have a real advantage in having almost no operating costs and low living expenses, which allows me to charge much lower fees than most people in my line of work.

The skills I use in my business are largely self-taught. I acquired these skills through my own initiative, outside of formal education.

Earlier this year, Michelle took a part time job in town. It pays well, provides some benefits, and brings her into contact with new people, which she loves.

None of this is making us rich monetarily, but it pays the bills, and meets our financial needs.

Aly entered college in this same period. She paid for her first year through scholarships and work, and has just paid for the coming term. She's signed a couple of student loans, but not the higher interest ones we hear about on the news. She has already begun to pay them back.

So yes, my family is better off now than we were in 2009.

But...

I should point out that we took possession of "the homestead" during the housing crash that occurred under the previous administration. We paid off both the old mortgage and the new one, so we never faced any problems with housing debt.

We survived the financial crash. It did reduce our retirement savings, but we weren't really relying on it.

And, incidentally, we never qualified for any of the special tax rebates that "everyone" got back then.

We looked after our own interests. We eliminated debt. We pared down expenses to a minimum. We get much of our food from our own efforts rather than paying someone else to provide it. Our jobs offer services that enough people want or need even in a bad economy.

In other words, we're not the kind of people who expect or demand that the President of the United States make things "all better" for us. The president isn't responsible for whether we succeed or fail, *we* are. Yes, some policies affect us directly, but for the most part our own efforts dictate whether we survive or go under.

So, perhaps we should ask a follow up to The Big Question: "If not, *who's fault is it?*"

Originally posted on The Zeiger Family Homestead Blog September 26, 2012.

LIVING SIMPLY

Simplicity is perhaps the most important aspect of our attitude. Simple living, for us, means doing without a lot of things that most Americans feel are essential to quality of life. It means finding pleasure and goodness in the everyday, the humble, and the unostentatious. True, we have many luxuries, many modern conveniences, and a fair few unnecessary toys by world standards—we make no attempt to be paragons in this regard! We just seem to be a lot happier with much less than most Americans have, or want.

Simplicity may be best defined as the ability and willingness to find satisfaction, contentment, and pleasure in the ordinary. If we felt no enthusiasm for what we own and where we live, if we could not entertain ourselves by our own resources, we would go crazy out here in the woods. While we always have much to do, time would eventually weigh heavily on us here if our temperament weren't suited to the life.

Acquiring simplicity may be easier than explaining it; I spend a lot of time writing about the concept, trying out different ways of describing what I think it is, and what it means to us. I guess I have yet to discover a simple way of expressing it....

The Key to Simple Living: Appreciating the Present

Our Christmas season ended last night at midnight. We have now returned to the every day. This in itself seems reason for celebration.

I've been struggling with terminology that expresses my current outlook on life. I like the phrase "celebrating the ordinary," but it has a more common use than my personal meaning.

The wider use of the phrase refers to the recent American tendency to elevate the mundane to special status, such as graduation ceremonies for advancing from one elementary school grade to another. I oppose this sort of thing. When I talk about celebrating the ordinary, I'm talking about enjoying the small features that make up a life, and enrich it—*if* we're paying attention.

Last weekend I heard a phrase on the radio that may express this better: "appreciating the present."

So, it's with an appreciation for the present that I transition from the Sacred to the Profane, from the Christmas Season to the every day. I've put away my special Christmas mug, and am enjoying coffee from my chunky white "every day" mug. I'm a bit more relaxed now that I'm not feeling the need to make the most of the season. It's a rather refreshing limbo, for the moment. I welcome the return to non-season-specific music on the stereo. I'm looking forward to starting a new book this afternoon, after I get out and cut some firewood. In the moments before I choose that next book, I'm enjoying the unlimited possibilities of what it might be.

These are small pleasures, hallmarks of a simple life. They aren't enough for most people—if they were, what a different world this would be! For me, the ability to appreciate what's going on at the moment seems like heaven on earth. Sure, I worry about the future; sure I strive to improve my lot. But in doing so, if I can maintain awareness of the good that's all around me, no matter how mundane, no matter how humble, I'll be a happier man, and perhaps a better one.

Originally posted on The Zeiger Family Homestead Blog January 7, 2010.

Sacred Coffee: Elevating the Habitual to the Mindful

Lately I've been considering the problem of habit.

For me, habit becomes problematic when the things I like to do become so ingrained that I do them without thought, thus diminishing my enjoyment, the very reason for doing it in the first place.

Specifically, I'm talking about coffee.

I love coffee. I generally have just one cup a day, because I don't need the caffeine, and because it's expensive. I consider it a luxury in our mostly subsistence lifestyle, far from coffee growing latitudes. I'm the only one in the family who drinks it, so it's a particularly selfish indulgence. I had assumed that I would need to give it up as soon as we moved here, but—thankfully—I haven't had to...yet.

Despite its special status in my life, I often find myself draining a cup with a certain amount of surprise. All of a sudden, the coffee's gone, and I wonder where it went. Immediately, I want more. I feel like I've been cheated of the pleasure of that first cup.

I'd been thinking of other things. My mind wandered elsewhere as I drank automatically. Only when I discovered that I'd finished the cup did my attention return to it. The coffee wasn't totally wasted, but almost.

Ironically, I've practically turned the coffee making process into a ritual. I take joy in selecting beans, particularly on those rare occasions when I splurge, buying from my favorite Alaskan roasters instead of purchasing Costco bulk beans. I love to grind beans by hand in my antique coffee mill, to carefully load the grounds into my Italian espresso maker, and to judiciously adjust the stove flame. I adore the smell of the brewing coffee filling the cabin like morning sunlight, and the burble of the coffee maker. After a ceremony like this, drinking the coffee without being fully aware of it approaches sacrilege.

For these reasons, I've concentrated lately on paying more attention to each cup of coffee. In fact, I've decided to consider coffee a sacrament.

Don't get uptight—I'm not proposing blasphemy. I'm thinking of sacrament in terms of an act set aside from the ordinary, to be performed or observed carefully, focusing on the act itself with appreciation and reverence. In other words, to *act mindfully*.

I see this as slightly similar to Native American tobacco use. I understand that many Native cultures elevate tobacco from the everyday to ceremonial status. What is for the vast majority of smokers a habit, often done with little or no awareness, is for these nations a sacrament. That's similar to what I want my coffee to be.

I still want coffee to accompany other pleasurable activities—reading, writing letters, listening to music, visiting—because coffee enhances them and vice versa. I just want to be more aware of the coffee while I'm drinking it, to be mindful of each sip, to taste and savor it. I want to know how much I've had, and how much I have left.

In my experience, considering coffee a sacrament wouldn't be so far fetched. I've sleepwalked through my share of church services. And I must confess, I've never felt the desire to go back and recapture the experience like I do a cup of coffee. For me, the latter is often far more satisfying than the former. Perhaps it's not such a stretch to consider it personal sacrilege to drink coffee without proper attentiveness?

Starting at coffee and extrapolating, I see many other activities in my day that require the same mindfulness.

Large or small, they deserve to be sacralized. The joys and pleasures of life can be celebrated as they come, or they can slip unnoticed into the background—performed, consumed, and attended to with little notice of what's happening, of how it affects us, or how it changes us.

As these joys and pleasures pass unnoticed, so pass our lives.

Originally posted on The Zeiger Family Homestead Blog November 22, 2009.

Simple Living: Simple Celebrations

Living a simple life, doing without most of the amusements and distractions our society finds so useful, not to say fulfilling, often means making one's own fun.

On our homestead, largely decoupled from the breakneck pace of the modern world, the rhythm of life is set primarily by the seasons, and their continuous cycle of holidays and observances.

We observe the standard holidays and family birthdays, of course, but these are augmented with minor holidays, anniversaries, and commemoration of personal milestones.

It's important to note that we don't do this to try to fill our days, to give our lives meaning and structure. We have plenty of that. We do it because we enjoy it, and have more time to do so than most people.

In this trivia-mad age, it's not hard to find lists of minor holidays, odd or historically significant anniversaries, and other days of note. We pick and choose among them to suit our interests and amusement. We celebrate Ben Franklin's and Thomas Jefferson's birthdays, because we admire these men, but don't concern ourselves with, say, Millard Fillmore's birthday. We flesh out the standard holidays with additional observances. The best example of this is the Christmas season, during which we observe Saint Nicholas Day, Saint Lucia Day, the Twelve Days of Christmas, and more in addition to the commonly observed dates in the season.

We also mark anniversaries of family milestones, such as the day we moved to the cabin. And, we mark a lot of days that are just plain trivial, even silly, like International Talk Like a Pirate Day.

We don't make a huge deal of most of these celebrations. For most, we make a nice dinner, our preferred celebratory method. Still, as we progress through the cycle of the seasons, the accompanying cycle of observations enriches our lives, providing the slight excuse necessary to celebrate, laugh, and enjoy ourselves.

Originally posted on Self Reliance Works November 27, 2011.

Living Naturally

Humankind is, of course, one with nature. Unfortunately, most us forget this, regarding the natural world as something other than ourselves, from which we stand separate.

If our family felt that way, it's very unlikely we would ever go to the effort it takes to live where and as we do. But because we embrace nature, and choose to live in it, we have become closely aligned to its rhythms, its demands, and its wonders. For us, living simply embodies living as one with nature.

Attuning to Natural Rhythms:
"Livin' by the Moon and Tide"

"It's another fine day across Mud Bay / Livin' by the moon and tide!"

—Burl Sheldon, *Another Fine Day*

Homestead life is very different from my former occupation. I pursued a broadcasting career for 16 years. That work required to-the-second timing. The ballet of synchronization became so ingrained that I still dream about it, years after my last air shift.

Now, we're attuned to natural rhythms, far more reliant on them than on clock time. My life runs on daylight and tide. I still wear a watch to help in planning, to keep us on time for concerts, meetings, and daily radio programs, and to satisfy curiosity. But I'm far less reliant on it now than in my former life.

To leave our peninsular home we must cross Mud Bay. The bay is shallow, but a small creek running through it creates a low spot that gets flooded by the tide.

The tidal range in our region can be more than 25 feet. We choose our tide and walk, or cross the bay by boat.

We can cross fairly directly in calf-high rubber boots up to a 13-foot tide, although we find 12 feet a more convenient marker. Anything higher requires hip boots, which gives us another foot of depth or so, or a hike around the head of the bay.

Hiking around is a poor option. It takes longer. The tidal meadow is a favorite haunt of bears and moose in summer. Winter cold makes it miserable.

Waves can build up in the bay, making it unsafe to cross by boat.

Tides aren't consistent across the entire range, but they're predictable. We use tide tables and "the rule of twelfths" to pinpoint crossing parameters. The rule divides the difference between high and low tide into twelfths, then uses that value to predict the height at each hour within the range.

We also use tide-plotting software that shows the curve of the tide, over which we can lay a marker at any desired height. Laying the marker at 12 feet shows us the times we can most conveniently cross in the tidal range.

These methods provide a general time frame. Actual water levels vary within the plotted range depending on conditions. Southerly wind raises the level of the flow, or slows the ebb. Rain and snowmelt runoff swell the creek above predicted levels. We keep a weather eye out, and adjust our crossings accordingly. We also rely on our knowledge of the terrain, crossing at points that offer different advantages depending on tide and current. Mistakes can mean boots full of ice-cold water, and soaked "town" pants.

The transition has been wonderful from timed-to-the-second work to "livin' by the moon and tide," as my neighbor, Burl Sheldon sings. Our current conditions are certainly harsher, more exacting, with potentially deadly consequences, but I wouldn't trade them for any other lifestyle in the world.

Originally posted on The Zeiger Family Homestead Blog November 13, 2009.

Simple Living: Attuning to the Seasons

Living on a homestead in Alaska is definitely a slower lifestyle, not because it's any less busy or full than others, but because our time is marked not so much in hours, minutes, and seconds as it is by the tides, the sun, and the seasons.

We have adopted the old Celtic or natural calendar, observing seasons from a different point of view than the modern way. The astronomical calendar starts a season on the day its defining feature changes (announce the start of winter when the days start getting longer? *Why?*). In the natural calendar, the seasons, as with all things in the world, don't spring full-blown into being, but start as an infant, grow to adulthood, then age and die, making way for the birth of the next season. In this view, then, winter begins November 1st, spring begins February 1st, summer begins May 1st, and autumn begins August 1st.* These season-starting dates make sense if you live in the northern part of the world, and are paying attention! On the homestead, we do pay attention. It's hard not to when we spend so much of our time outside. At our latitude, each seasonal shift is apparent around the dates given above. The changes can be somewhat subtle, but we watch for the signs, because our livelihood, even our lives, depends on an awareness of the changes. We're different from most Americans, who only need to look

---

*Christian readers may notice that this is the calendar that drives the pagan observances. People who live in harmony with nature rather than contempt ("this world is not my home...") will, of course, be far more attuned to the changes around them. Of course, this same calendar led to the Christian holidays being placed where they are.

up from their dashboard or desk and notice that, on December 21st, the "first day of winter," the season is fully upon them. We need to be better attuned than that. And, I would argue, because we are, our lives are far richer than most people's.

Originally posted on Self Reliance Works November 20, 2011.

Living By the Season: A Meditation

People talk about living more deliberately, being more self-sufficient, decoupling from the breakneck pace of the modern world. We believe in that, which is why we're here on the "homestead." We live not by the time clock, but by the weather, the tides, and the seasons.

This is on my mind a lot just lately, as autumn is probably our most transitional season. This is the time of our year when activity increases, yet we prepare for and look forward to winter, the slowest time of year. Activities that we've pursued through the summer, like gardening, foraging, fishing and finding firewood intensify as we harvest the planting, more wild foods ripen, the fish run, and cooler weather dictates that our wood stove, which has remained largely unused through the summer, is once again called on for heat.

These activities will peak soon. The wild harvest will end, mostly, with the first freezes and snows, which usually come in early November. Mushrooms are wiped out then. Most of the berries will be gone, although some, like highbush cranberries, crowberries, and nagoon berries, will improve with a frost, but could be hidden by snow. We have planted our cold frames, and can reasonably expect a few greens to continue growing through the winter.

Wood gathering will improve through the winter, both because the hot work of bucking deadfalls and splitting is easier in the cold, and because snow allows us to sled the wood home rather than carry it.

The fish are theoretically always available, but they're not as abundant in the winter, nor is it safe to pursue them from ice-coated rocks or from wind and human-powered small boats on storm-tossed waters.

The winter will turn us inward. We'll still get outside virtually every day, but we'll spend more time indoors on quieter, less strenuous pursuits. The holidays will come. Neighborhood gatherings will increase, promising potlucks, excellent food, fellowship, and saunas. It's a good time of year, one we look forward to as we make this last push.

Anticipating the coming lull of winter makes the transition a bit more difficult. While cool, clear autumn days invigorate us, the wet, cold, windy ones make it all too easy to practice for winter. We sense the urgency to store up, to sort out and stow seasonal clothing, to winterize everything we can, to prepare for harder weather, but we are seduced by another cup of coffee, tea or cocoa, one more chapter in the book, that one really good song playing on the CD or radio—anything that would keep us inside by the fire for just another minute or two....

In this, our fourth autumn on the homestead, there's consolation in experience. We know that it will not all get done. We also know that some of it will get done not in autumn, but in winter, or even spring.

The blessing of the seasons is that they are cyclical—what passes will come again, both the opportunity and the need to complete the task. We will finish projects; some will need redoing when the season rolls around once again, others will be done for good and all. New projects will be added to the list next year. Worrying will not change that. The cycle continues, and life abides.

Originally posted on The Zeiger Family Homestead Blog October 3, 2009.

Opening Up to Nature

A reader recently commented on last year's post about our homestead anniversary. Her request for advice on how to create a life similar to ours, and my reply, got me thinking on the subject, and led me to expand on it further here.

The most important part of the reply as far as I'm concerned, was my recommendation to not wait for the home(stead) of one's dreams before beginning to live the lifestyle to the desire and extent possible. Jenna Woginrich provides the best example of that in her wonderful book, *Made from Scratch: Discovering the Pleasures of a Handmade Life.*

Further, though, if one longs to live in partnership with what I like to call "Big N Nature," it's all around us, available to be appreciated by us, and to nurture us, if we're willing to let it.

This sort of thing has been on our minds lately, as Aly prepares to go to college. While her campus features acres of undeveloped forestland, and offers a fairly wild setting, it is adjacent to what is, to our lights at least, a fairly large city.

We look on her new life as being far more urban than the one we enjoy, so we tend to think of her as about to become less integrated with nature.

However, we forget that even in the biggest cities, the wild creeps in. Wildlife, from songbirds to coyotes and deer encroach on the most urban landscapes. "Weeds" flourish to the point of becoming problematic. These creatures and plants are largely invisible to most urban dwellers, but to anyone open to seeing them, they're quite visible.

I still strongly advocate getting out of the big cities to enjoy Nature more fully. Obviously, we would think that way. However, it's trite but true that one can "bloom where one is planted." After all, that's what Nature is doing. If you're a part of Nature, why can't you?

Originally posted on The Zeiger Family Homestead Blog August 17, 2011.

Attitude Adjustment through Animism

On a summer day, a friend and I stood on the cobble beach of Mud Bay, pulling crabs from the floor of my canoe and butchering them on the rocks. I worked silently, focusing on not getting hurt by the crustaceans' powerful pincers or by their sudden shrug that might smash my fingers against the sharp shoulder spikes.

My friend talked to the crabs as he worked, cursing their attempts to fight him, laughing at and taunting them, describing what he planned to do next, and the cooking process to come.

To my surprise, this shocked me—not only because it struck me as disrespectful, but also because it interrupted something I had been doing without even thinking—silently addressing the crabs myself.

I mentally apologized to each crab for treating it so cruelly, and thanked it for the food it would provide my family and guests. I behaved like an Animist, treating the crabs respectfully as sentient beings, even as I killed them.

I didn't try to explain this to my friend—that would not have gone well. I merely suggested, mildly, that the crabs fought us for their lives, and shouldn't be blamed for it. And, I silently apologized to our arachnid victims for my friend's disrespect.

On a winter day, Michelle and I stood in the forest above our cabin, surveying a grove of trees. We needed straight, limbless poles of sound, fresh wood for a building project, and had chosen these trees to fell for lumber after the winter's cold made them dormant. We had laid our plan long before, in early autumn, and our minds had been made up to harvest the trees. Still, I hesitated. I couldn't bring myself to cut down these living trees, my companions since first coming to the property, my silent protectors and company as I worked around them in the forest. To cut them down seemed a betrayal of a friendship.

"Praying" to crabs? Friendship with trees? Yes. I also thank the fish I catch and the birds and animals I kill for food. In short, I act like an Animist.

Having been raised Christian, I'm culturally conditioned to find this sort of behavior silly or naïve, perhaps even contemptible, as you likely do as you read this. I "know" that plants are inanimate, and that "lower" life forms are nearly so. But I've come to think of it differently than I was taught.

And, significantly, I don't do this for *them* so much as I do it for *me*.

I find that by treating with respect the plants and animals that I use to sustain my family, I remember to use them responsibly. An inner monologue of thankfulness orients me toward treating them as if we truly had a relationship—which, I would argue, we do.

After all, I depend on them for our survival and quality of life. By addressing them as sentient beings I find that I'm more careful to kill as quickly and painlessly as possible when necessary, and to do so only when necessary. I also try to clean and prepare them well, to reduce waste as much as I can, to use every part of them possible. Regarding them as fellow creatures to whom I owe respect changes how I regard the raw materials I derive from them.

The Christian answer to this is, of course, to thank God for the benefits we receive from these plants and animals. That's fine, but then, perhaps it's not the whole point. This practice tends to objectify the plants and animals as something given to me by an other, rather than reminding me that they are living things, with instincts or inclinations to continue living that are assumably every bit as compelling to them as mine are to me. Giving the respect and thanks to a creator god inserts a remove from the affected creature; respecting the entity itself reminds me of what I owe to it directly for ending its life. Use implies responsibility. Gratitude engenders respect.

Scoff if you like. I don't expect this explanation to change anyone's way of thinking. I benefit directly from the practice by being more careful about how I use these resources. I also feel better for it.

Originally published on The Zeiger Family Homestead Blog January 31, 2013.

Foraging: Finding Food for Free!

We are a family of hunter/gatherers, with definite emphasis on gathering. We forage or "wild craft" a lot, harvesting food, herbs and seasonings, tools, even medicines from the land and sea around us. It is one of the biggest "jobs" we have on the homestead.

In their season, we harvest mushrooms, berries, seaweed, legumes and vegetables, tree buds, and medicinal herbs. Throughout the year we harvest mosses, seashells, cones, and shelf fungi. A lot of our "hunting" is actually foraging, since gathering seafood from the beaches at low tide hardly qualifies as a hunt, even though the end product is meat for the table rather than vegetables. In a wider sense, we also gather inorganic materials from the wild for food or building, such as sand and gravel. In fact, we even forage snow!

Wild foods and medicines are so prevalent that we have trouble keeping track of all that's available, what it can be used for, and when. The list is overwhelming, the subject of many books, and every plant seems to have myriad uses. They're all around us; many of them are literally at our feet.

This creates an interesting dilemma in garden planning. Michelle and I disagree on what should or should not be cultivated. I maintain that we needn't grow domestic foods that can be found growing wild locally. Why grow peas when large patches of beach pea line our coast? Wild plants need not be tended, so cultivation efforts could be focused on foods that do not appear naturally in this area. Michelle maintains a small plot of indigenous plants on the edge of our garden, both for decoration and to ensure that specific ingredients are at hand when needed. It's her garden, I just weed there, so I can only grumble about it.

Wild crafting requires study, careful observation, and an awareness of the seasons—both in the regional sense and the local year-to-year variations. The window in which a plant is useful may be quite narrow, so timing is extremely important, as is the ability and willingness to get out and gather when the gathering's good!

Right now, the gathering's good for mushrooms. This is one of the last harvests of our year, until the snow falls, but that will be detailed in due time. If you follow this blog, you'll eventually learn about a wide variety of harvests on and around our little homestead.

Foraging not only provides free food and other benefits, it has aspects that make it a part of our spiritual life. Wild crafting creates in one an awareness of the seasons, a respect for the land and its bounty, and a connectedness to nature that is sadly lacking in western society. The process of finding and harvesting wild edibles drives us outside into the weather, among our wild neighbors, many of whom compete with us for the foods we seek. Foraging not only feeds our stomachs, but in many ways, it feeds our souls.

Originally posted on The Zeiger Family Homestead Blog September 29, 2009.

"Hunker Down" Days

This morning, as I do every morning, I walked out into the teeth of the weather in my pajamas. We, like generations of Americans before ours, have a "little house," an outhouse.

For most contemporary Americans such a thing is unthinkable. For us it's a very real connection to our environment. Looking out the window to *see* what the day is bringing you can't compare to getting out into it half-dressed to *feel* what it's bringing you!

What I felt today was a Hunker Down Day.

Here's the deal: every day we ask ourselves, "what will (or did) I do today that will sustain this lifestyle?" It's an important question. Other than maintaining a handful of investments and micro incomes, most of our time and energy focuses on keeping us clothed, fed, sheltered, and warm. So, what did I do today? Did I gather firewood? Did I catch a fish? Did I work in the garden? It's important to move ahead, not to get complacent and fall behind.

Then there are days like today. The wind is somewhere around 30 knots and it's raining heavily. These are fairly common conditions in Southeast Alaska, even in our area, where it's a bit drier than the rest of the region. On a day like today it's not difficult to get outside, but it's the kind of day when you look for indoor projects that allow you to sit down, enjoy a cup of coffee or hot cocoa. A project like updating the blog perhaps....

Some days are best declared Hunker Down Days, although we've learned to be very cautious about such declarations. Just like the last administration's ridiculous color-coded threat assessments, such a declaration can quickly get out of hand.

The first winter we spent on the homestead was a pretty tough one. It was the harshest winter any Haines old timers could remember—and our old timers have a lot of winters behind them! The schools closed for an unusual amount of time. Irresistibly drawn to the allure of an honest-to-goodness snow day, even at our age, Michelle and I were quick to decide that if her public school peers weren't studying, Aly didn't have to home school that day, either. We would observe these snow days in solidarity with the townsfolk. With several feet of snow in the dooryard, freezing spray dashing in from the wave-torn rocks, and the wind howling above 45 knots, it was a Hunker Down Day if any deserved the term.

So we snuggled down in front of the wood stove, hot drinks at our elbow, to read or play games, or perhaps write letters.

Then a funny thing happened. Of course, we couldn't tear our eyes from the windows. The storm proved more exciting, and more comprehensively plotted than most television shows. Soon Michelle noticed the weirdly shaped hollows the wind had carved around every unmovable object. Our curiosity grew, and before long we bundled up and went outside to strap on snowshoes. We had to climb the trail up the ridge behind us, the trail that leads eventually to the bay, and then to the road.

What we found is hard to describe. Imagine, if you will, a steep wooded slope, over which tons and tons of refined white sugar, or perhaps foam, had been poured. Then, in mid flow, it suddenly congealed. The wind, baffled by cliff faces and slopes, swirled through the forest, sculpting the snow. It was breathtaking! We decided that since we were out, we should hike as much of the trail as we felt like, breaking the new snow to preserve the track.

We knew what could happen: one night Michelle hiked out for a community meeting. She was gone only two hours at most, but when she returned, the piling and blowing snow had erased all trace of the trail.

Luckily, she knew the way well enough to make it home, but we learned the wisdom of repacking the trail now and then.

Snowshoeing is a pretty good workout, and by the time we turned back toward home, we'd covered more than three-quarters of the trail. We arrived home hot, winded, and flushed.

So much for hunkering down.

True, we weren't really working, but we had accomplished something, and, as far as recreation, it was a lot more strenuous than working on a puzzle or shuffling a deck of cards.

This is just one example. I have observed that a declared Hunker Down Day almost always guarantees more work will be accomplished that day than on a "regular" day on the homestead. Either the weather improves unexpectedly (which often happens) or restlessness sets in, or our attitude changes after a couple of hours of rest and relaxation. Perhaps more significantly, I suspect that by giving ourselves permission to take it easy for a day, we remove the pressure to be out and doing, and focus switches from the *obligation* to achieve to the *pleasure* of achieving.

Because I've learned an important lesson. Actually, I think I've always known it, being raised this way, but I've proved the lesson time and time again living on the homestead: not all work is work.

Working for the good of one's family, on projects that make a better life for yourself and the ones you love is not the same as working for wages. Yes, the ends are the same—working a "real" job earns the money to spend on family needs, so the effect is much the same.

But, having worked most of my life at a strange variety of jobs, none can compare to the satisfaction of the work I do now. Working at making a living for yourself and your family is more than work; it's prayer, or meditation, maybe even recreation in the most literal sense of that word. It's much more physically challenging than the office jobs I used to have, but at the end of a day on the homestead, I think I'm less tired than I ever felt after a calm day at the office. Maybe the tiredness I'm talking about is spiritual, not physical.

I see a couple of important differences between these two types of work.

First, our kind of work is self-scheduled. We work our own hours, at our own pace. If something more important (or even just more fun) presents itself, we switch to that. Or, we knock off for a while, to see a whale go by, or to bird watch, or snack.

Secondly, we do it as a family. This is not to say that all of our projects are worked on together. Most are not. But we have access to each other. If Aly has a question for me, she knows where to find me. She doesn't have to call the office, and have a receptionist or the voice mail tell her that Dad's busy and can't take her call. If Michelle finds yet another large rock in the garden, she can summon me to help pull it out. If a neighbor drops by to visit, we can stop what we're doing and sit down to chat over a cup of tea. These are the things that make work a pleasure, rather than...well, a job.

Another lesson I've learned is that while it is important to move ahead, to make progress on ensuring our continued existence here on the "homestead," the whole thing won't come tumbling down if, every now and then, we hunker down.

That is going to prove one of the most important lessons learned here. We do have to keep our eyes on the prize, as it were, but we don't need to create stress over it.

To do so would jeopardize the whole plan. Little by little, things will get done.

This is a hard lesson for me. As head of the family I feel a responsibility to ensure our survival. But I am beginning to see that my perception of what should happen, and when, is not the best plan.

For instance, accumulating firewood seems like a no-brainer: obviously, the woodshed must be filled with enough wood by mid-autumn to see us through the winter. But in reality, this may not be the best, safest course. While the vision of a huge pile of wood, dried, seasoned, neatly stacked, stored up against the ravages of the coming winter is overpoweringly seductive, it is far more sensible to focus my energies elsewhere, and accumulate that supply of wood more slowly. It doesn't make sense to be up in the woods on a warm day, sweating and bug-bitten as I buck up a fallen tree, when the salmon are running past the rocks. The tree will still be there a month or two later, the salmon won't. A month from now, the bugs will be gone, the days will be cooler to the point where a good vigorous workout with a saw would be welcome. There may even be snow on which to sled the rounds down to the cabin for chopping.

If I reject the ideal I've conjured for myself and attend to each task in its proper season, I lessen the work and discomfort of one job, and avoid missing the window of the other.

So, the Hunker Down Day is there for us when we need it, but, like most treats, it must be doled out carefully. You never know what might come of it.

Originally posted on The Zeiger Family Homestead Blog September 25, 2009.

LIVING FRUGALLY

Living on our homestead, we've turned the American dream on its ear. Rather than working hard to make enough money to acquire belongings that display our status to our neighbors, we've stripped down our expenses and expenditures to the minimum possible, adjusted our lifestyle to live within those means, and set to work for ourselves, focusing on performing the tasks that keep us sheltered, fed, and happy.

To do this required a lifetime of frugality and attitude, most of which we owe to our parents who raised us as they did. The essays below provide a handful of the many examples to be found on the blog of our attitudes toward material belongings and acquisition.

"Think Little"

I recently read Wendell Berry's excellent essay, *Think Little,* from *A Continuous Harmony: Essays Cultural and Agricultural.* Berry's thoughts and suggestions in this piece, and the observations of other thinkers and authors, have helped crystallize my own thoughts about the point of view that influences the way my family lives.

The concept of Thinking Little may be considered another expression of simple living, but with a slightly more clarifying emphasis.

Berry suggests that the American motto: "Think Big," should become "Think Little." He urges us to change the way we conceptualize what we need or want, to turn away from seeking the biggest, the best, and the most of everything to pursue only what works best for us.

I can hardly think of a better illustration of this concept than Boletus Edilus, the king bolete mushroom we hunt in our forest at this time of year.

Arguably the most delectable mushroom, I've described the bolete's qualities previously. Part of what makes this mushroom more precious is its transience. It is a favorite food of flies and other bugs, some of which lay eggs in the fungus. These develop rapidly into tiny maggots that consume the 'shroom from the inside out. Often, maggots will infest a bolete before it even breaks the surface of the soil.

At the same time, boletes can grow to huge proportions. The amount of mushroom flesh a forager may find varies markedly as a tiny button grows to a full grown mushroom. The question becomes, how big can it get before the insects that seek it as avidly as the mycologist corrupt it?

On rare occasions, we find large boletes that the bugs have completely missed. We've found fresh specimens large enough to feed two people.

However, because the insects are so common (and because they never sleep) we have to fight against our American desire for the biggest and the most. Our best strategy is to harvest whatever we find as soon as we find it. We dare not leave a good bolete for even an hour. If this means settling for less mushroom, so be it.

"Settling" may not be the correct word. While we may miss out on a sense of pride or triumph from finding a massive mushroom, the small, freshest boletes are far better than the more mature specimens. Their flesh is as firm and crisp as a young turnip, and their flavor is superior to their elders. A smaller but better bite seems best.

As with boletes, so too with other aspects of our lives. Perhaps not the latest fashions, but good, sturdy, reliable clothing. A good, useful car or truck will almost always serve far better than a luxury car. While enough money can provide a certain level of security, massive amounts seem to create problems, possibly even dissatisfaction.

Here on our "homestead" we tend to Think Little. We'll touch on this theme often in the future, I'm sure.

Originally posted on The Zeiger Family Homestead Blog August 28, 2012.

Develop Healthy Attitudes Toward Your Belongings

I adhere to the principal that happiness comes not from owning what you love, but from loving what you own.

Compared to most Americans we have very little; what we do own we take pride and pleasure in. We try hard not to take any of it for granted. At the risk of overusing a common buzzword, we try to use our possessions mindfully.

Luckily for our income's sake, we have simple tastes. Michelle has never been very interested in jewelry. Our clothing tends toward practical rather than fashionable. In fact, we tend to rebel against "fashion" in many ways. We don't keep up on the latest trends. Neither do our neighbors, which helps considerably.

Our tastes in belongings are also simple. I take great pleasure in particular styles of eating utensils, such as forks and spoons, mugs, and wine glasses. My favorite fork and spoon styles are commonly carried by cut-rate cafeteria suppliers, and can often be found in thrift stores. My odd little collection of other peoples' castoffs gets used more often than the name brand flatware Michelle and I received as a wedding present over 30 years ago. I have two particularly favorite mugs. One was a gift from my brother, the other I found in a thrift store. Our sturdiest, most trusted dishes are inexpensive Corelle Ware®. Even our precious and beloved "winter" wine glasses are, we eventually discovered, from a fast food chain premium campaign!

No doubt all of these things earn us the scorn of our "betters." In college I remember a wealthier classmate disparaging Corelle Ware®, which I'd used ever since they became the "new dishes" in my parents' household. Luckily, her sort of person never seems to make it out to the homestead for dinner, no doubt saving them much displeasure and discomfort. We don't seem to feel the loss of their company, ourselves.

I can't lie and say we wouldn't like to "trade up" on some of our possessions. We're human, after all, and not wholly separate from our consumer-oriented society. However, these feelings are rarely strong enough to act upon. If something wears out, we replace it if we must. If we find an excellent bargain, we might replace something early, especially if we can sell the old item, store it as a back up, or give it to someone who really needs it.

And yet, we're happy! How we manage that without constantly consuming new and better goods is a mystery. I suspect a certain level of self-satisfaction may be a factor.

Another key to our happiness is being able to let these possessions go when necessary.

I have always felt that transience enhances beauty and value. Flowers are more beautiful for their brief life; the joy of a bunch of balloons is enhanced by the shortness of their duration (this is why I find mylar balloons unpleasant—they last too long!). Soap bubbles are even more precious, being so much more temporary. Good food must be enjoyed when fresh.

I try to apply this same aesthetic to possessions. We must handle glassware delicately to preserve it. Breakage is to be expected—doesn't the very fragility of a fine-stemmed glass enhance its beauty?

Many of my personal treasures are rare; should they become damaged or lost, it's very unlikely they could be replaced. I consider them even more precious for that reason, rather than holding out hope or expectation that they might be restored somehow if necessary. If they are lost, I try to focus on remembering the joy they gave me when I had them, rather than mourning their absence. I try to say "I had it once" rather than "I'll replace it." In the few cases where I have actually replaced an item, I found the replacement inferior to the original, as it lacked the pleasant associations of the first. The replacement is a mere reminder of the lost article's significance.

The possible exception to this is books, and perhaps movies and music. Such items, where the content is key, can be replaced, although particular editions of books— especially ones gifted by special friends—are more difficult to restore.

By cultivating this attitude, we've managed to transition more smoothly from "normal" American life to a far richer, more rewarding life on the homestead. The necessity of padding our nest egg with as much cash as possible, and the daunting task of carrying everything we owned to the homestead, spurred us to sell as many belongings as possible before the move. Eventually, we donated a considerable amount of goods to charity. Accepting transience in possessions became key to making a successful break, and has continued to help us maintain an excellent lifestyle on very little money and no steady income.

It's certainly not for everyone, but how does one know until one tries? It needn't be all-or-nothing—but small steps in the right direction could eventually lead one on an incredible adventure!

Originally posted on The Zeiger Family Homestead Blog October 28, 2009.

Want To Save Money?
Set Your Standards Too High!

Quite unwittingly, I've stumbled upon an excellent frugality measure: idealism.

I love *stuff*. This doesn't mean that I have a lot of possessions—at least not by today's standards—but I really like the things I own. Each item represents a successful search for the right object, whether an essential tool or knick-knack. Each one has been weighed against others of its kind, and judged superior. I rarely buy anything without considering quality and cost.

This isn't because I'm extremely frugal, it's because I'm an idealist! Quite often when I want or need something, I'll create an image in my mind that represents everything I want that object to be, then I'll search for it, stubbornly refusing to accept anything less.

The likelihood that my ideal image may not exist at all is key to the frugality. If there's no such product, I can't buy it!

I love snow globes, but I don't own a single one. Years ago I developed an image of what I'd like my snow globe to be: the shape and size of the globe, the scene depicted in it, the particulars of the base, and most importantly, no bubble in the top of the globe! With this ideal firmly in mind, I shopped for years without success. I got a lot of pleasure from the search, and enjoyed seeing many beautiful snow globes in the process.

About ten years later, I found a globe that met all my qualifications. It was beautiful, as perfect as my vision, and it was extremely affordable. Oddly, though, by that time, it just didn't seem like something I needed to own right then. I turned away from the opportunity. Years later, I still have no regrets! I guess the long search cooled my ardor for the object.

Some years ago I found a mug in a gift shop. It had a beautiful design sand blasted through the glaze, but I especially liked its graniteware finish and wonderfully heavy construction. I admired its size and the way it fit my hand.

It cost $30! I began searching for a better price. Four years later, I found one selling for $8. For the next three years, I decided to buy the mug each time we returned to that town; every time, I decided against it at the last minute. The next summer, I found a mug of the same design, without artwork but in a far more pleasing color. It was in a thrift store. I paid $1. It is now my primary coffee mug. In fact, you can see it on the cover of this book.

I have a mental list of objects I want or need but don't own, because I've yet to find my personal paragon. Each one represents savings, as I've never spent the money for it. These ideals have given me almost as much pleasure from the search as I would derive from ownership.

Originally posted on The Zeiger Family Homestead Blog October 27, 2009.

Museum of Lost Desires

Haines has one of the best secondhand stores you could ever want. Owned and operated by a friendly proprietor who really only does it to entertain himself in the off hours of his real job, caring for his aging parents, it is a treasure trove of ever-changing, capital S *Stuff*.

The store may or may not have an official name. It might be "The Garage Sale Store," but most seem to call it for its owner, simply "Ralph's."

I love going there. We find a lot of things we need at prices we can afford; Ralph's fun to visit with, as are the other customers, many of whom we know, some we've come to know after sharing a comfortable conversation among strangers in Ralph's shop.

There's a particular reason, though, that I appreciate the store. For me, it's a Museum of Lost Desires.

I recently returned to the store after a long absence. Aly and I found a few things we needed, but I enjoyed the other items even more. I found many things that I once had a keen interest in acquiring, but never got around to doing so.

I love stuff, which makes it hard to be frugal. But, browsing The Garage Sale Store reminds me of just how far I've come.

That day I found a fancy, Italian style espresso maker that I'd seriously considered buying once upon a time, just before settling for my stovetop espresso maker (also Italian, but far less intricate and expensive than the item I'd considered). Finding the machine at Ralph's would have been a huge score, as whatever he was asking for it would be a fraction of what I would have paid for new back then (I didn't even look).

I also found a mug that I'd once wanted rather badly, although not enough to buy it. The shape of it, and the drink it advertised (recipe included on the side of the mug) appealed to me once. I'd forgotten all about it until I saw it on the store shelf.

There are several shaving mugs in the store. When I began using an old-fashioned shaving brush, I searched for a mug much like these. Ralph's prices are affordable, unlike what I found during my search. Since that time, I've settled on a plastic ware container that, while not as pretty and stylish as an antique shaving mug, does the job better, and can easily be sealed for travel. Michelle wanted me to choose one of the mugs as a gift from her, but I declined—they're beautiful, but I honestly don't need one anymore.

The list goes on. Every visit reveals desirable objects from my former life. It's nostalgic and somewhat bittersweet. Mostly sweet, as I am reminded of how many times I've foregone a purchase, and realize how little those acquisitions would mean to me now.

Originally posted on The Zeiger Family Homestead Blog April 10, 2011.

We have a tradition of buying Aly a Christmas ornament every year, so that when she starts her own home, she'll have a collection of treasures with which to decorate her own Christmas tree.

Christmas 2012, I found a little ceramic ornament at The Garage Sale Store that Aly and I had admired there on the day that inspired the post above. I purchased it as her ornament for that Christmas. Besides the meaning its shape represents to Aly personally, it is now also a reminder of pleasant hours rambling through Ralph's crowded, eclectic little shop.

Make Your Belongings Last—
Read The Instructions Often!

Resistance to reading instructions is so pervasive that I needn't bother belaboring the old jokes. Who doesn't approach a new tool with the certainty that they know how to operate it without reading instructions? And, who among us who bothers to read instructions hasn't become totally exasperated by the condescending tone, uselessly obvious warnings, and ubiquitous English-as-a-foreign-language garbling found in most instructions?

The fact remains, though, that if you want full, proper, and extended use of a tool, it's important to read the instructions. Further, it's important to *reread instructions periodically!*

Recent memory studies reveal uncomfortable evidence that we only remember something once. Afterward, we remember our *memory* of the information! This implies that any errors in operation can compound and multiply over time. For this reason, I'm trying to train myself to periodically reread instruction manuals.

This is also important because of our disposable society. No matter how frugal we are, we inevitably cycle through a series of goods, each with slight differences in the proper way to operate them.

I learned this with coffee makers. I use Italian style stovetop espresso makers, and have owned three of them through the years. Each one had its own recommended heat setting. I no longer remember which coffee maker requires which setting. I ensure longevity and proper use of my current coffee maker by periodically consulting the instructions. I find this particularly helpful, since the current one requires the least care—I'm constantly reminded that I'm actually being too careful with it!

The instruction manual I consult the most is the one for our wood stove. It's vital that this stove last as long as possible; it's the first we've ever bought new, it suits our needs perfectly, and we paid far too much and worked way too hard to bring it to the property not to ensure its use for many years to come. I read the sections on cleaning and maintenance, and on building and maintaining a proper fire about once every six months.

This exercise never fails to recall some important detail to my memory. Failing to consult the instructions would lead to incorrect use of the stove, very likely shortening its useful life.

These two examples inspire me to be meticulous about reviewing instructions now and then for all my belongings. This is especially important for expensive, complex machines, like an automobile. It may just be the most common sense frugal practice I follow.

Bottom line: it's your stuff. If you don't want to replace it often, learn how to use it right, and periodically remind yourself of how to do so.

Originally posted on The Zeiger Family Homestead Blog October 15, 2009.

When "Good Enough" is Best

In general, it makes sense to obtain the highest quality tool you can afford or find, whenever possible. However, many times "good enough" beats "best." The trick is considering all the angles before making your choice.

After yet another knuckle-busting bout of changing out the propane tank, I decided the time had come to give in and buy a proper-sized box wrench for the job. I'd been limping along with my adjustable wrench, a geriatric tool that has developed a tendency to loosen its setting during use. I've been watching garage sales and second hand stores for more than a year, hoping to pick up a used wrench in the proper size, but I finally decided to buy new.

I shopped around town, finding one wrench for an alarmingly high price, and another for 1/3 that price.

If someone handed me both tools and asked me to choose for free, I'd take the more expensive one. I judged it to be a superior piece of equipment, one that would probably last longer than the other. However, for the price, I could "risk" purchasing the other, inferior wrench. If it broke, rusted, or otherwise wore out, I could buy another one like it and double whatever time I found it useful, and still save money over purchasing the better tool. In this particular instance, where the tool is dedicated to one specialized use, the "good enough" tool will likely last longer than I'll need it.

I learned this strategy from my older brother. When I started building sailboats, I considered buying a top-of-the-line circular saw. My brother suggested I buy a cheaper model of lesser quality. He predicted that it would likely last long enough to do the job, but if it burned out, I could buy as many as three others like it before paying the same amount as the one top-of-the-line model's price. That was more than 10 years ago. I still use that first "good enough" saw. Since then, I received two others like it at no additional cost when we bought the homestead. The gamble paid off in this instance as well.

Perhaps I'm missing the satisfaction of owning the best tool for the job, but I find saving money on "good enough" pretty satisfying as well.

Currently unpublished.

In Praise of Pack Rats

The man who built our homestead is a master pack rat, a quality that I greatly admire.

When he and his family moved away, everything they left behind came with the property—and they left a lot behind. Not a week goes by that we don't bless them for something; usually, it's for squirreling away items of value that we find we need.

I try hard not to buy something I need until I've made sure there aren't any here already.

One evening, a neighbor and I worked together on one of our gas generators. When he asked if I had a certain tool, I told him I didn't know. He remarked that it was the kind of tool any homestead should have. In my defense, I said, "I probably do have it, I just can't lay my hands on it right now. In all likelihood, I have seven of them in the shed."

I checked the next day, and I was wrong. I actually have ten of that particular tool—not seven!

The shed is a treasure trove of previously used items, waiting to be put to their intended purpose, or adapted to new ones. Often, when I go to town in need of something, I recognize it when I see it—I've already got some in the shed. Other times, someone will show me the manufactured item I'm looking for, but will then tell me that I could make the same thing for less. Once they show me the needed components, I'll realize I've got them all in the shed. If they explain how they go together, I can go home and make them myself out of what I have on hand.

I built all the connector cables for our battery bank this way, without needing to purchase any components.

My favorite example of this came when we decided to build a new, cantilevered tower for our wind generator. I needed a 20-foot length of schedule 40 steel pipe to make a tower that accommodates the generator's mounting sleeve. When I priced this, my jaw dropped!

I decided to think it over. I knew of several lengths of pipe around the homestead that were long enough, but I discovered that they were smaller than the required diameter. However, in the shed, I found a 3-foot section of schedule 40 in the correct diameter. I quickly discovered that it fit perfectly over one of the other pipes—I merely needed to drill them, slide one over the other, and bolt it into place to make a tower top of the correct diameter. My cost: a couple of bolts to secure it. In addition to the cost savings, I avoided the chore of carrying 20 feet of steel pipe to the homestead.

Part of the pleasure of benefiting from this horde of items is the as-yet unexplored potential. I have an amazing collection of doohickeys, designed for purposes I have yet to discover. Who knows what I could build with what's on hand?

The mind boggles!

Originally posted on The Zeiger Family Homestead Blog March 26, 2010.

"Abusing" Credit Cards to Add Value

Michelle and I are "deadbeats," and proud of it!

Credit card companies refer to cardholders who pay their balance in full every month as "deadbeats." Paying in full avoids interest charges, which represent most of the card issuer's profits. A "good customer" in their view is one that consistently carries a balance, accruing interest.

Living a mostly subsistence lifestyle with no steady income, you'd think we'd be strictly cash-and-carry. Actually, credit cards form an important part of our financial strategy.

Americans are caught in the credit web. The system is designed to draw us into debt and ensnare us for life.

Like it or not, a major credit card is almost a necessity in this society. Major credit cards are considered better personal identification than government-issued I.D., including driver's licenses. That's so wrong, but it's true!

We use credit cards to "abuse" the system. Most credit card companies offer some sort of premium— often a rebate of 2% or more of one's annual spending.

If one has self-discipline—and that is absolutely vital to success—these premiums represent added value. To get the premiums, we charge every purchase we can, always paying what we owe at the end of the month. Obviously, this requires that we limit spending to available funds.

We use credit cards for very specific uses. We try to buy locally, but some items we need just aren't available. In the Internet age, purchases are most convenient with credit. Our most active card accrues frequent flier miles on our regional airline. It takes a while to earn a free ticket at our rate of spending, but it represents significant savings. The required spending exceeds the cost of a ticket, but we receive other goods and services for that expenditure—the ticket's a bonus.

Some merchants offer discounts for paying cash. Credit transactions are a burden that most businesses are forced to bear for fear of losing customers. We try to help when we can, but are even more likely to do so when there's an added advantage to us.

Maximizing benefits means remaining flexible and vigilant. If there's any threat of increased fees or decreased premiums, we complain. If benefits don't exceed fees, we ask for a lower level of service in return for no fee. We hardly need most of the "benefits" cards offer, just the lowest level that provides premiums.

We've held our cards for years, and the companies seem averse to losing us. Often a call to customer relations changes the agreement to our advantage. If not, we will simply cancel the card, since it's no longer benefiting us. We show no mercy, expecting none from a business that labels a customer who pays what's owed when it's due a "deadbeat."

Originally posted on The Zeiger Family Homestead Blog March 5, 2010.

Eating Garbage: Making the Most of Our Food

I had an odd realization a few weeks ago. My family was eating dinner. Most of our focus and effort was on the meal, although one or the other of us surfaced briefly now and then to remark on the meal's deliciousness. We were all full, but we couldn't resist seconds, perhaps even thirds, because we couldn't stop savoring the flavors. How incongruous, then, to suddenly realize *we're eating garbage*.

I'd best explain immediately. Our meal was turkey soup. This meal arose from the remains of our Christmas dinner, when Michelle simmered the "frame," the skeleton of our turkey on the wood stove most of a day. She added spices, herbs, and homegrown vegetables, and let it cook some more. Finally, she added some dumplings. The resulting meal is fit for a king!

So where does the garbage come in?

Consider:

- Americans throw away at least 40% of their meals every day!
- Many Americans will not eat leftovers at all!
- Our homegrown vegetables—perfectly sound, wonderfully nutritious—aren't pretty enough to pass physical inspection in your local grocery store.
- Except for the herbs, spices, and flour for the dumplings, everything in our soup would be garbage in most American homes.

Many Americans turn up their noses at leftovers. We even know people like this personally—luckily, I can't recall whom at the moment, or I'd "out" them on the

Internet right now. Even the venerable turkey dinner, lauded for its production of leftovers, is in reality barely used at all before it's thrown in the garbage. A day or two of sandwiches at best, and it's out of there. Some few go so far as to make soup, but far too many do not.

As for the vegetables, for most of us, they come from the grocer, not from the ground, and they'd better be picture perfect, or it's no sale. Bruised, blemished, slightly less than classically shaped, and they're relegated to the dumpster out back.

That's a sad, sobering realization. This soup is so good, it's like eating dessert for dinner! It fed us for two nights. It would have gone three, maybe more, if we could have controlled ourselves, and not gotten greedy about tasting more and more of the excellent flavors.

But here's one more detail: this batch of soup was the second one Michelle made with that turkey frame. She'd already made one batch from it, which fed us for 3-4 days. This soup came from *leftover leftovers.*

This isn't an isolated case. All of our meals are like this—most of them generate leftovers that will be used in a variety of ways until they're completely consumed. We have no refrigerator or freezer, so occasionally food spoils or gets contaminated by rodents before we eat it, but we work hard to avoid that.

Michelle's an excellent cook, but she's not a miracle worker. Anyone could make a soup as good as this with very little training, skill, or effort. All it takes is a willingness to eat the wonderful, bountiful food that most of us wouldn't even consider, other than as garbage.

Originally posted on The Zeiger Family Homestead Blog January 25, 2010.

FAMILY

Perhaps no desire compelled me to pursue this lifestyle more than wanting to be present as our daughter, Aly, grew up. I abhorred the concept of leaving the family every weekday to spend the bulk of the day working outside the home. I wanted to be a part of what happened each day, rather than hear about it after I'd found my way home from work. The greatest blessing of our life on the homestead has been working, playing, laughing and loving as a family.

Space and Time Enough for Family

Since my youth, I've loved reading stories set before the early 19th century. In many of them, if the owners of a large house, particularly one situated out on the moors, decided to throw a party, that implied that their guests would be invited to move in with them for a month or more. A Christmas "party" could mean a giant sleep over through the whole season! This seemed to be the fashion because these estates were remote, and travel to them was a difficult, dangerous undertaking. It also suggests a less-hurried life, more conducive to long, pleasant associations.

Compare your last planned visit with family or friends to one in which you would have weeks of uninterrupted time with them. "Visiting" would cease to be an obligation that must be attended to properly within the limited time available. It would stretch out into long afternoons and evenings of conversation or companionable silence. There would be space for time alone, time for various groupings among the family, ample opportunity for meaningful interaction. Visiting would become communing. Scheduling would become meaningless beyond agreeing when to get together for meals, games, or outings.

This brings to mind the concept of "family," a word that for me has a much larger meaning than some people might be willing to accept. I believe in blood ties, and the importance of the nuclear family, but I also accept that families can be built as well as born.

Families can be created by bringing together people who love each other, whatever their ancestry or associations. Each traditional family begins, after all, with

the marriage of two people who are not related. Doesn't
it stand to reason that the same bonds can be formed in
larger groups? We can adopt grandparents, uncles, aunts,
children into a family, can't we?

If this seems strange, consider my upbringing: I have
had four grandmothers and five grandfathers. My
mother's family accounts for the extras. Her parents
divorced. My grandfather remarried and my grandmother
acquired a common-law husband. When my mother was
in high school, she stayed behind to continue school
when her family moved away. The couple who housed
her and cared for her during that time, making her a
member of their family, became my grandparents when I
was born. After I grew to adulthood, my blood
grandfather passed away, and his second wife, every bit as
much my grandmother as any in the bloodline, eventually
married again. The wonderful man she married became
my grandfather. While I regrettably have not had the
opportunity to get to know him well, he is my grandfather
through the power of my love for my grandmother, and
her love for him.

I have several aunts, but the one I know the best is
my mother's half sister—a technicality that has no
meaning to me whatsoever. She is my aunt, and I don't
love her any less for our reduced blood tie. I know her
better than my other aunts because she came and lived as
a member of my family for two extended periods when
she was a teenager.

After all, other than similarities in looks and
temperament, how does blood enter into it? When I
learned that men and women I called "Grandma" and
"Grandpa" were not actually related to me, that was a
curiosity, but made no difference to my feelings for them.

My example isn't even that extreme. I've known
many excellent families where the relationships are
untraceable.

Perhaps this is why I'm especially touched by books and films that describe a wider concept of family. There's Rat and Mole's extended cohabitation (before moving in on Badger) in *The Wind in the Willows*, and the film version of *Under the Tuscan Sun*, in which Frances answers an accusation that a young man who works for her has no family by saying, "That's not true. He has me. *I'm his family!*" The film *Cold Mountain* presents one family forged from the tatters of several in the aftermath of the American Civil War. These and many other stories impress me with the myriad possible family configurations that extend beyond the man-woman-children model without losing meaning or value.

Perhaps the only requirement is that one's heart be open to the possibility of finding and accepting people worthy of love.

Feeling this way, imagine how wonderful it was to find the "homestead" we now own, a compound complete with a small guesthouse. I immediately saw the potential to live out my childhood dream: the buildings may be small, but there's room to pitch tents on the grounds if necessary, room to spread out and relax together. There's a common area upstairs in the main cabin that can fit extra sleepers. There's room—room for family.

In the years we've been here, we've had some good family visits. Some of that family can claim blood ties, others claim ties of affection. Some of these visits have been almost long enough. We haven't achieved our full potential in this regard, but we're ready to make it happen should the opportunity present itself.

Because, as the First Rule of Family dictates: "There is always room."

Originally posted on The Zeiger Family Homestead Blog November 8, 2009.

The Importance of Family Meals

More and more studies lend truth to what many of us consider common sense: sitting down to family meals is important to developing and sustaining family and community ties, and promoting education, health, and wellbeing. Such an idea seems obvious, but in our society, it apparently isn't.

A friend told me about a Sunday service once where his pastor asked for a show of hands of those who regularly sit down as a family for evening meals. In a congregation of 100-200, his and one other family raised their hands. Sadly, my friend's family consisted of him and his wife—no children. Many Americans just don't sit down to family meals anymore.

Of the many reasons this is detrimental to society, two glaring ones stand out: it degrades family cohesiveness, and it leads to poor eating habits. "Grab and go" fast food meals replace healthier sit-down dinners, if a meal is eaten at all.

Eating individually, or with friends robs families of a time to reconnect with each other, to talk, share, plan, laugh, cry, and love. All of these vital moments in a family's life are all too often usurped by schedules, commitments, even a desire to avoid the family moments!

It's far too easy for me to talk about family sit-down dinners. I have a rare advantage over most Americans in this regard. We are a one-child family, and we live in a remote location, so dinner doesn't compete with other activities. However, this was far from true when I was a teenager; and yet, my parents maintained family meals.

In high school, my brother and I were very active in extra curricular activities, many of which threatened to encroach on the dinner hour. My parents seldom had to insist that we eat at home as a family, but they did when they had to. I remember several commitments that needed to be rescheduled, because the Zeiger boys would not be able to participate without rescheduling.

The key to bringing your family together for meals does not lie in insisting on it, because that has the opposite effect. Requirement leads to resentment. Better to cultivate a need within family members to gather. Here are a few suggestions:

- Let everyone know that there will be a favorite dish prepared for dinner or dessert that night, something you know they won't want to miss.
- Whenever the family gathers, focus on making it a good time, so that everyone will be likely to want to do it again. (Don't force this!)
- Keep the door open to guests; if your children would rather spend time with friends, bring those friends to your table and your children will follow!
- Make family meals a priority for yourself, and honor that priority. If you won't, who else will care?
- Whenever you can corral them, try to keep them. Unplug the phone, turn off the cells. Leave the television, radio, and computer off. Limit distractions, so that family is more likely to turn to each other for entertainment.
- If you must, institute a weekly dining out night. If you can't gather them around the home table, gather them at a restaurant.
- If all else fails, negotiate one night a week for a family meal. Most schedules can allow at least one night at home "penciled in."

- Be consistent. In time, everyone will come to expect and depend on these family gatherings, and will make sure nothing interferes.

No doubt you have some ideas of your own. Try it—your family will be better for it.

Originally posted on The Zeiger Family Homestead Blog April 9, 2013.

Reading Aloud to Your Family

The Zeiger family has a favorite activity that entertains, enriches, educates, improves self-confidence, and brings us closer as a family: we read aloud.

We started reading aloud before we could properly be called a family. It played a role in Michelle's and my courtship.

One afternoon on our college campus, I laughed once too often at the book I was reading. Michelle had asked each time what was funny, and I'd read her the passage, until finally I returned to the beginning and read the whole book aloud. This very pleasant shared activity soon became a habit, particularly during long car trips. It's very convenient to read a book in which we're both interested together instead of individually.

Both of us are avid readers. When Aly arrived, we raised her as one of us. Besides reading to her regularly from children's books, we included her in our oral reading.

We didn't worry about the complexity of plots or prose, trusting her to comprehend as much as she could. In this way, she first heard Richard Adams's classic, *Watership Down* when she was 4 years old. She adored all of the story's richly layered facets. If tension mounted, she cuddled close and helped pull the rabbits through to safety.

Once we realized that she could follow the story through pages of adult prose and over many evenings of reading, we never worried again, other than perhaps to edit on the fly occasionally if the action took a particularly age-inappropriate turn. We tried not to "pull punches," and made sure to stop and discuss when necessary.

This led to some very meaningful family exploration of issues that everyone must face eventually. I'm sure it led to Aly's ability to think critically about hard issues, to assess and express her feelings, and to weigh consequences.

We still read aloud, even though Aly is now a teenager, and a fast reader. Some titles are ones she's read, and has asked that we share. If it's new to her, she inevitably rereads it (sometimes repeatedly) after we finish.

Behaviorists cite reading aloud as key to child development. It stimulates an interest in learning to read, facilitates the process, and teaches by example. From our experience, we feel everyone involved benefits, not only from the books we choose, but from the family activity itself.

Most of our reading falls to me. As a former broadcaster with a fair amount of acting experience, I enjoy performing. Also, since reading aloud requires us to be together, and the listeners like having something to do, I manage to get out of a lot of cooking and dish washing this way!

If you don't read aloud in your family, you ought to give it a try. It's not hard, and doesn't require any particular skills. You don't have to be perfect, just consistent—the minimum requirements are that you can read and speak loudly enough to be heard by your family. So what if you stumble? Who cares if you can't "do" voices (which I generally avoid)? All that matters is that a family voice shares a good book with the assembled listeners.

The more you do it, the better you'll become. If you can't learn, grow and improve in the bosom of your family, where can you do so?

Some members of your family may resist group reading initially. Don't insist on participation. Far better that it be voluntary! Gather everyone who *is* interested, and give it a go. Human beings thrive on storytelling. Before long the reluctant ones will likely be drawn into listening in spite of their best efforts.

Here are a few things to keep in mind while reading aloud:

- Choose a time when you're not likely to be interrupted, or rushed by upcoming events.
- Make sure everyone's comfortable.
- It helps if everyone has a quiet activity to do while listening (hint: handheld video games and other electronic devices don't count!).
- Be aware that some of these activities may require occasional discussion. Don't insist on total quiet while you read. Allow interruptions when necessary.
- Keep an eye on your audience. Quit if someone starts to nod off.
- Don't overdo it! It's easy to get carried away with the story and wear yourself out.
- Never insist that anyone read to the group. This is an activity people should look forward to, not dread.
- Make sure the reader has sufficient light for the task.

Keep in mind that reading aloud is not the same as reading to one's self. It takes longer, and should be allowed to do so. Don't rush—spend the time the book and your family deserve! Savor each phrase, reading for meaning rather than to "get through it." Reading aloud is a leisure time activity, not a job! Relax, enjoy yourself, and don't worry about making mistakes. You'll do just fine, and your family will love it.

Originally posted on The Zeiger Family Homestead Blog November 6, 2009.

"Pioneer Night": Making Conservation and Emergency Preparedness Fun

When we lived in Juneau, we developed a tradition that is so ironically juxtaposed to our current lifestyle that when friends remind us of it, we're momentarily stumped. The tradition provided an excellent weekly break from "normal," helped us to prepare for emergencies, and saved money. We called it "Pioneer Night."

Juneau is prone to power failures. Outages that could last from an hour to days disrupted many an evening's plans. We took these in stride, switching to other activities; the main crisis involved finishing any interrupted cooking. We had a wood stove for heat, and a few flashlights, candles and oil lamps for light.

We noticed that we often felt a bit disappointed when power returned. The novelty of an outage appealed to us in some way. A minor crisis must be overcome; our activity became more family-focused without computers, housework, or music to distract us (television was rarely a factor, as we'd canceled cable years before). We gathered close to the wood stove for warmth, and talked. Sometimes we'd play games, or make music. Restored power signaled a return to a normal that seemed less appealing than the preceding "emergency."

This led to "Pioneer Night." Thursday evenings we turned off heat and lights, started a fire (if needed) and lit the house with oil lamps and candles. We ignored appliances; we even avoided opening the refrigerator if possible.

We prepared meals accordingly. Soup or other hot meals from the day before provided easily reheated leftovers. Sometimes we'd have salad, or cold finger foods—crudités, bread, and slices of cheese. Eventually, Michelle experimented with cooking full meals on the wood stove, unwittingly laying the groundwork for our future lifestyle.

We ate sitting on the floor at a low, round table near the fire. Occasionally we played wind-up music boxes for ambiance. After dinner, I usually read aloud while Aly and Michelle played or worked on hand crafts.

We arranged our collection of oil lamps throughout the house, wicks trimmed, reservoirs filled, and matches available for instant use. No need to rummage in the dark for lamps or candles. Our emergency lights became incorporated into our décor, and weekly use habituated us to their location, maintenance and operation.

The custom provided a weekly reminder of the value of ready-at-hand electricity. It also taught us we could manage well without it when necessary. We noticed a 25% drop in our electric bills through this and other small conservation measures.

"Pioneer Night" soon became a source of spiritual and mental refreshment. Like most Americans, we longed for weekends. Thursday's change of pace through Pioneer Night felt like extra time off.

Our experiment in conservation may seem frivolous, but perhaps not. On October 21st, 2009, utilities in Anchorage and Southcentral Alaska conducted a two-hour test of natural gas conservation. They asked residents to lower thermostats and hot water heaters, and postpone washing dishes and clothes. Participants reportedly reduced consumption by about 3%. I've not heard participation estimates, but I wonder if presenting it as a Pioneer-Night-like event might not have tempted more people to get involved?

Friends, some of whom have established their own "Pioneer Night," speculate that we're now living it 24/7.

Ironically, this isn't so. Since we generate our own power, electricity's cheaper than lamp oil! True, we do cook on the wood stove a fair amount. Our décor still features oil lamps and candles, ready for emergencies. "Pioneer Night" served us well, even after it became, for us, a memory from a former life.

Originally posted on The Zeiger Family Homestead Blog October 26, 2009.

Stupid Fun

If you are a frequent reader of this blog, you may be justified in thinking that we take life pretty seriously around here. Most of the posts seem to be about the work of the homestead, or maintaining its finances, or Aly's studies.

I'm proud to say that, while we do apply ourselves to all these things, we also understand and practice the art of having stupid fun.

Recently, we sat on the rocky cliff of our beach, dangling our feet over the edge. Our harsh weather has softened, warming up to the mid-40s with light winds and sunshine. We enjoyed the warmth of the sun on the rocks around us. The water, far below us at that tide, seemed crystal clear. We could easily see bottom, and enjoyed the play of sunlight on it as ripples in the water warped and rumpled it.

Aly remarked that she really wanted to throw rocks. Michelle got up to return to the garden boxes she had been building, but before leaving the beach, she returned with a double handful of rocks. Aly offered to share them with me. Never one to pass up the chance, I accepted, and we happily splashed away for a while.

When the rocks had been used up, we contemplated the water for a moment. Then Aly said, "I wonder if we could pry up the lumps of spray ice over there?" I could think of only one way to find out....

Soon we were working together to lift big slabs of ice, some over 6-inches thick, and heave them into the water. They created huge splashes. If they didn't shatter on impact, they plunged beneath the surface, then bobbed back up in a hugely satisfying manner. Occasionally we'd stop to rest, examining the odd little bits of things embedded in the ice—tiny mussel shells, a barnacle or two, algae—and tasting the ice to see if it was salty or not (it's not). Then we'd be back at it again, hurling ice chunks into the water and watching them float away. At one point a sea lion popped its head out of the water like a disturbed neighbor, to see what we were doing.

We weren't accomplishing anything. We weren't improving our lot, or helping others, or earning our keep. We were just having stupid fun.

And you know, it felt pretty darn good.

Originally posted on The Zeiger Family Homestead Blog March 27, 2011.

Unschooling:
Self-Directed Learning on the Homestead

Aly crouches on a windswept beach, carefully steadying a digital camera. Below her, a family of river otters chuckles and pipes to each other as they swim past. She adjusts her headphones, listening as an otter dives near the hydrophone she has suspended in the water. Aly is unschooling; the world is her classroom, and school is always in session.

Unschooling, developed by educator John Holt and advocated by Grace Llewellyn, particularly in her book, *The Teenage Liberation Handbook: How to Quit School and Get a Real Life and Education*, is the most common sense approach to education we've encountered.

Unschooling recognizes that humans are self-teaching creatures, perfectly capable of learning anything they need to know without institutionalized education. In fact, our education system often depresses the natural ability to self-teach, and discourages a love of learning! Unschooling advocates unstructured, self-directed learning through experience, personal inquiry, and exploration.

We began home schooling when we moved to our homestead.

Initially, Aly's years of institutional learning shaped her expectations of education. She learned to be passive, to wait to be told what to learn and when, and how to proceed. It taught her that homework is drudgery, and that grades are the only way to assess progress.

Institutionally educated ourselves, Michelle and I were little better: much of the transition from schooling to unschooling involved breaking free of our perception of "the right way" to teach and learn, and open our minds to a better path to education.

Now in her fourth year of unschooling, Aly takes the initiative. She knows that no one else will do it for her. She's moved beyond institutionalization and has achieved self-direction, becoming skilled in seeking and finding answers to her questions.

Michelle and I have had to suppress our pedantic tendencies. Holt warns against trying to teach your children, stressing that any subject, no matter how interesting, immediately seems less alluring if a parent suggests it! Taking a hands-off approach, allowing Aly to pursue her own interests has been very difficult.

We've devised strategies for sharing knowledge in subtler ways. We've become adept at initiating conversations on specific topics, addressing each other rather than her. If there's a book I want her to read, I'll read it and talk enthusiastically about it at the dinner table, discussing why I liked it, rather than why I think she might. If it interests her, she'll pick it up. The times I forget and make a recommendation, or bring something to her attention, she often won't follow up. On rare occasions, if I think she'll benefit particularly, I'll break the rules and assign work. We will always teach her to a certain extent. That's our privilege and responsibility as parents. We're always ready to answer any questions she cares to ask. We'll explore topics with her. Mostly, we go about our business, and hope that she takes an interest in what we're doing. Thankfully, she often does!

Unschooling works best when parents are engaged—facilitating, not leading. Children raised to have self-discipline, a spirit of inquiry, and an ambition to achieve their goals will succeed in unschooling. One must be self-directed in life to successfully direct one's learning!

We're all engaging in self-directed learning here on the Zeiger "homestead." The learning curve is steep, and new challenges must be faced as they arise, often without the luxury of researching them beforehand.

Originally posted on The Zeiger Family Homestead Blog October 20, 2009.

Aly graduated from Mud Bay Home School in 2011 (first in her class!). In the spring of 2013, her second year of college, she qualified as a Junior, and continues to work toward a degree in her chosen field. The preceding essay introduced the topic of home schooling on The Zeiger Family Homestead Blog. As our most important priority, Aly's education became a major focus on the blog. You'll find many more essays on her progress there, including her graduation, the various programs she found to participate in, and how her test scores and other achievements helped prevent our local high school from being designated a "failed school" through the No Child Left Behind Act.

.

The Real Value of Homemade Gifts

The phrase "homemade gift" can strike fear into the stoutest of hearts. We all act as if they are a good thing, but if hard pressed, relatively few people honestly want to receive, or to make homemade gifts. I think we see them as requiring more talent and effort on the giver's part, and more grace on the receiver's part, than most of us feel we possess. Even so, I'm a fan of giving and receiving homemade gifts, as long as there's no requirement to do either.

I firmly believe that homemade gifts are best when voluntary rather than compulsive. Our family places no restrictions on gifts; if an item is needed or wanted, we procure it if we can. If we can make it ourselves, that's excellent, but it doesn't have to be homemade.

While every Zeiger family Christmas includes some homemade presents, certain gifts stand out more than others, such as the year I built Aly a working toy trebuchet. My gifts to Aly this year [a pair of wooden drop spindles, revealed on the blog after Christmas day] show promise of being particularly special, and as I worked on them I thought more about this value.

Simply put, making gifts connects the giver and the receiver more than a purchased gift could.

Most of us have experienced the joy of finding the perfect gift for a loved one. An appropriate gift, found at a bargain price, can be wonderful. The anticipation of seeing the person receive the gift is keenly felt, and should not be discounted.

However, a person who comes up with an idea for a good homemade gift for a loved one, plans the process, and executes it, spends all of this time and effort for the receiver. Necessarily, the person the gift is intended for—created for, as that term cannot be emphasized enough here—is central to the giver's thoughts, hopes, and concern throughout the creative process. The act of making a homemade gift is a meditation on the loved one destined to receive it.

This is why making homemade gifts gives me such joy. Even in the darkest moments, when the materials have been cut incorrectly, or a bad slip has damaged a perfect piece, or the glue or paint dries too quickly, too slowly, or not at all, it is for the benefit of someone I love. The person for whom the gift is intended becomes a constant presence. I find myself barely able to bear the wait for Christmas morning, when I can give the gift, and share the experience of making it: the inspiration of it, the stories of success and failure, tidbits of information about the object's history and use I've learned in the process.

I really believe that the person giving a homemade gift benefits more than the person receiving it. Which may be why I do my utmost to make the gift as well as I can.

Making gifts for Aly has been even better since she went away to college. The downside of making gifts, for me, is the necessity of secrecy, the need to separate myself from the receiver to accomplish the work. This year, I managed to finish [the spindles] before Aly arrived home. Every moment of working on them brought me closer to her at a time when we were unavoidably absent from each other. I didn't have to tear myself away from her to finish the job! That's taught me the importance of planning these things well.

Originally posted on The Zeiger Family Homestead Blog December 19, 2012.

The drop spindles are another example of frugality, an aspect of homemade gifts that I did not include in the post above. Because I used recycled materials, and tools and supplies I had on hand for other projects, I only needed to purchase a 4-foot dowel to make the spindles. Each shaft came close to 12 inches, and the dowel cost under $2.00, so each spindle cost less than 50¢ out of pocket.

RESOURCE USE

Perhaps one of the most startling realizations we have experienced since moving to the homestead is that modern conveniences are often merely that—conveniences.

Conveniences are not necessities, although they become regarded as such in a surprisingly short time.

None of us are so many generations removed from the time when outhouses were common; both of my parents, and my father-in-law used them growing up. Both indoor plumbing and refrigeration, now regarded by most Americans as absolutely essential, are still unknown in much of the world in the 21st century. We've even discovered the elegant utility of hand tools and other devices that were perfected generations before we became a civilization driven by the convenience of cheap energy.

As Americans, our whole existence revolves around instant applications of heat, electricity, and water at a thoughtless touch. For a few, like us, this is no longer true. Amazingly, this proves to be less of a problem so much as a reawakening to possibilities.

The essays that follow address our new paradigm, in which modern conveniences give way to different, more satisfying ways of living, and precious resources are used wisely.

Life Without Refrigeration

As outside temperatures creep upward from the low teens we've seen lately, our food is migrating once again, from the bedroom windowsill back to the cool box.

We have no refrigeration on the homestead. We use a shelved box set into the wall of our enclosed porch that is familiar to my parents' generation. I think it used to be called "the cooler," although in this modern age that term implies a plastic thermal box. The old fashioned cool box relies primarily on shade and air circulation to keep foods cool. In very hot weather, I imagine chunks of ice, purchased from the Ice Man, would be set on top of the box to help. In very hot summers, we use tubs of seawater and a canvas sheet. Draped over the outside wall, evaporating water helps cool the box.

Mostly, we simply watch for spoilage, buy small quantities of food, and use it before we lose it. We also adjust our eating habits seasonally, to lessen the need to keep leftovers or other perishables. Cooking always means heating thoroughly to prevent food poisoning, as we did even when we lived a "normal" life.

In winter, the opposite conditions keep us busy. Mostly, we enjoy longer shelf life for perishables. Pots of leftovers can be stored on the floor of the porch, with proper precautions against rodent invasion.

During cold snaps, the box won't insulate well enough to keep liquids from freezing. Anything left on the porch becomes a popsicle in short order. When that begins, we move food to the bedroom sill.

The cabin's master bedroom is an add-on to the original structure. The wood stove's warmth doesn't penetrate well there, and the less insulated windows allow the room to grow quite cool. Luckily, this is how we prefer to sleep: cold room, warm quilts. A jug of milk or other perishable, while not cooled to refrigerator temperatures, stays fresh for a long time.

In our modern world, we've lost sight of how long food can last without refrigeration. I remember reading a time scale printed on the back of a milk carton, and being amazed by the number of days milk could be expected to stay fresh at room temperature. When you factor in the margin of safety against litigation this display incorporated, the chart showed what a luxury a refrigerator actually is.

We have a variety of thermal coolers on hand for overflow. We sometimes fill the bottom with seawater to help cool food. Sometimes these also insulate food against freezing in the cold snaps. Our root cellar averages about 40-45° year 'round, so it's a good back up through hot summers.

I'm not advocating getting rid of your refrigerator, I'm only observing that the machine isn't as necessary to life as I'd grown up believing. If we could figure out a way to use a refrigerator here economically, we might consider it. Some day we might try one of the myriad cooling schemes suggested by friends and family, if we decide the results would justify the expense and effort. But for now and so far, we're doing okay without it.

Originally posted on The Zeiger Family Homestead Blog January 15, 2010.

Doing What's Necessary:
The Homestead "Facilities"

We're often asked an indelicate question: "How do you…um…?" Which obviously translates to "Where do you *go?*" Here on the homestead we deal with human waste with pit and composting outhouses.

Both our outhouses, for the main house and the guest/boat house, were pit-style when we moved here. The main house's hole was nearly filled, so we began a new plan immediately. We brought a composting toilet with us, originally purchased for a live aboard sailboat we planned to build. This may be an excellent toilet for our homestead…someday.

A composting toilet collects waste in a container of fine organic material, usually peat moss, where it is dried and mixed until it becomes odorless compost.

For optimum operation (and, it's a toilet! Optimum operation is *essential!*) this composter requires a warm room, and must be vented out the roof. Our outhouses are pretty much out of the running as candidates to house this machine. The boathouse outhouse's walls are only about three feet high, after which it becomes an open booth (which allows great views, by the way—of the mountains, not the occupant!).

The main outhouse is enclosed, but there are gaps between planks, and the door is half-Dutch: the bottom half opens, but there's no top half.

The door, incidentally, is a large, metal reflective sign that reads: "Danger: Explosives!" The original owners have a delightful sense of humor.

This building will need insulation before it can effectively house the composting toilet.

In the meantime, we've adopted an ingenious plumbing-free toilet, an inexpensive bucket-based composting method that works extremely well. In fact, we may never commission the commercially manufactured composting unit!

At one of the first potlucks we attended in the neighborhood, I plucked up the courage to ask the hostess about their outhouse strategy. I admitted my question might be an inappropriate topic, but she assured me that outhouses dominate "polite" conversation here!

In that spirit, I'm willing to "talk toilets," sharing with you—in frank yet discrete language—details of the compost system, secrets for improving performance, "the rules of the little house," and other observations on living with outhouses, including encounters with unexpected visitors.

Originally posted on The Zeiger Family Homestead Blog September 23, 2009.

Headed Straight Into Darkness

The old Tom Petty & the Heartbreakers tune has been running through my head these last few weeks, as we've passed through what Michelle poetically calls "deep autumn" into the infant weeks of newly-arrived winter. At the moment, we're losing daylight at a rate of five minutes a day. We are, as Mr. Petty et al sang, headed "straight into darkness."

Mental health professionals are gearing up for the annual Alaskan epidemic of seasonal affective disorder (SAD—seldom has there been a more fitting acronym!). They won't find me asking for help. I adore the darkness. I embrace the night!

Despite our free wind and solar-generated power, a generous collection of oil lamps, and an impressive arsenal of headlamps and flashlights, we use artificial illumination less often than we could. We've simply become habituated to less light. Usually, the normal coming of daylight is adequate. If not, we often begin our day by the wood stove's light and perhaps the oil hurricane lamp above the table. As long as we're not trying to read, the soft light of morning is perfect for lighting the room.

On these days we wear headlamps, which can be switched on for a moment to illuminate a brief morning task, then turned off.

Eventually, daylight fills our home, and we extinguish the lamps or candles.

Human eyes can adjust to darkness to a remarkable degree—far more than most Americans realize, being so used to lighting up darkness with every available watt.

I noticed long ago that using a light limits vision to that which the light can illuminate. Sight narrows down to the limits of the light, instead of expanding to take in all available natural light.

With a flashlight, one can only see what one is pointing it at, while blinding one's self to everything else around. Usually, it's better to have full peripheral awareness of shadowy figures than a bright illumination of a thin beam's worth of view.

This, and the practical matter of saving batteries for when they're really needed has led me to move around in the darkness as much as possible without lights.

"As much as possible" is an important qualifier. Humans aren't nocturnal—we require a little bit of light to see by. You would not believe how truly dark it gets here! Many nights our bedroom is so dark we can't differentiate between the wall and the window.

We see no artificial light other than our own, or on rare occasions, light from a passing ship. We occasionally see a faint glow from Haines to the north, if we're standing where we can see up the canal. Our view of the night sky is spectacular—we can clearly make out the Milky Way and other formations that are invisible to most town dwellers. Our view of the aurora borealis is excellent! If the moon's out, we often use no lights at all in the yard.

Our comfort in low light led to an interesting comment from a friend of Aly's who spent a week with us. After returning home, she told us she realized that she didn't need to turn her bedroom light on just because she'd entered the room—that there are plenty of times when she could see well enough without it. Her visit to our "homestead" freed her from a wasteful habit she hadn't even been aware of.

Life is easier and safer for us in the light half of the year, but the dark half also has its attractions and comforts. After so much time at one extreme, it's nice to return to the other as the circle of seasons swings around again.

Originally posted on The Zeiger Family Homestead Blog November 15, 2009.

Clothing: Essential to Survival and Self-Esteem

"Trust not the heart of that man for whom old clothes are not venerable."

—Thomas Carlyle

Clothing is one of the essentials of survival, along with food, water, and shelter. Western society's relationship to clothing is particularly complicated by the influence we've allowed it to have on our self-image. If we must, we can hide in a corner and eat unfashionable foods. Water, despite inroads made by designer bottled "varieties," is still, in essence, water. Even a home that speaks less well about us than we might wish it to can be hidden from those whose esteem we seek, as long as we look good in what we're wearing.

Clothing is a great concern to us on "the homestead." We are less fashion conscious than most— our main concerns are durability, comfort, and protection from the elements.

Living on almost no income, we face an interesting dilemma, that of finding the highest quality for the cheapest price. What we need to obtain must be inexpensive. What we have must last as long as possible.

Finding high quality clothing at rock bottom prices would be impossible, except that we're blessed to live in the United States, home of the most acquisitive and least frugal people on earth! The sheer volume of clothing that our nation casts off each day is unbelievable. Luckily for us, many of these rejects end up in thrift shops!

I got over the stigma of hand-me-downs at a very early age. Not only am I the son of a minister, I'm a younger brother. I worried about dressing fashionably, like any teenager, but I never reached the point where I rejected my brother's hand-me-downs, or the bounty of the church rummage closet.

Finally, I become attached to clothing for sentimental reasons, and rarely part with a quality item until it wears out completely. I have shirts that I've happily worn for 30 years and more.

My reluctance to pass on clothing led to storage issues in our home, which only resolved when we moved to the "homestead." Suddenly, my oversized wardrobe became an impressive stockpile of clothing. Boxes and boxes of clothes for all seasons fill our shed, some of which I won't open until the clothes I currently use wear out. So what if they're out of style? They weren't that fashionable when they went in the box in the first place. What do I care? Are they comfortable? Do they protect me from the elements? These are the questions that concern me. Like anyone else, I want to look good, but I think I do okay without being a slave of fashion.

Originally posted on The Zeiger Family Homestead Blog September 25, 2009.

Reduce, Reuse, Recycle

Reduce, Reuse, Recycle. I would assert that the three parts of this concept are listed in order of importance. If we want to save the planet, cut back on the tremendous rate at which we use resources, be they renewable or not, or simply improve our own personal lives, each of these three concepts must be pursued in the hierarchy indicated by their order.

Reducing what we consume obviously has the greatest impact. Decreasing the volume of goods we want and/or need sets a new threshold for consumption. Living at or below that threshold lowers one's cost of living and decreases the amount one must earn to maintain a lifestyle "to which one has become accustomed."

We've definitely found this true in our homestead life. As much as we spend on food and other necessities, and things we want rather than need, it's still drastically below the levels we spent when we lived "on the grid," as frugal as that life had been.

Recycling, which should be the last resort of these three concepts, has regrettably become the main focus. Even the triune logo has become known by the common name "recycling logo."

Recycling is very important to conservation, but it is the least effective of the three concepts. This is true not only because the process of recycling uses valuable energy and resources in and of itself, but because it is the most convenient of the three concepts, and is therefore the most favored. After all, recycling a tin can is still, as far as the convenience of the individual consumer is concerned, the same as throwing it away. It goes into a bin, just like garbage, gets hauled to the curb, just like garbage, and, just like garbage, gets picked up and dealt with by someone else—disappearing quickly and conveniently from one's life, with the added benefit of being better for the planet than tossing it in a garbage can.

Still, we need to recycle everything we can't otherwise use. It's far better than throwing it in the landfill. But anything we can reuse should really never be recycled.

Reuse comes between Reduce and Recycle. It may be the most important of the three. Every time an object is reused for its original purpose, or repurposed for some other need or want, the item's life is extended without significant additional processing. That means that a reused item uses far less time, energy, and resources than a recycled item. Whenever we find a new use for a manufactured product, or use it again for its original purpose, we do more for the planet, and our own personal finances, than we can through recycling.

Originally posted on The Zeiger Family Homestead Blog March 19, 2012.

Reuse Glass Before Recycling It

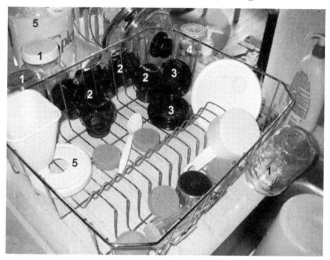

As I argued in the last post, anything we can reuse should really never be recycled. For instance, glass.

Consider: glass doesn't decompose. This means that if kept in a usable form (such as a bottle or jar) it will not wear out in many, many lifetimes. As long as it's kept unbroken it can serve its original purpose indefinitely.

This is why you find so many glass containers in old homes and ghost towns. Or, would, if collectors hadn't come through ahead of you and cleaned them out as antiques. This is also why I get in so much trouble with Michelle, because I try to hang on to as much glass as I can, against the day it might become useful.

She understands to an extent. She leads the charge in collecting and saving sound canning jars. These take pride of place in our storage areas, and more are always welcome. She's less understanding of my hoard of wine bottles, and I've given up on buying glass drink ware that catches my fancy in the secondhand stores.

Nevertheless, we try to keep as much glass as we can store, and put it to use. If we don't need it today or tomorrow, it'll still be ready to use years from now, for no more additional resource use than the water and soap to clean it.

The photo at the beginning of this essay illustrates this perfectly. I took it one day after removing labels from marmite jars. When I looked at it, I began to realize just how much reused glass the photo contains. In it, you see:

1. Canning jars. The quart jar has a plastic twist cap that is a handy alternative to the canning ring and lid for resealing after use.
2. Marmite jars. These will soon be filled with homemade salve. Their yellow lids can also be seen in the drainer.
3. Lids from a set of glass canisters. The canisters have broken. Aly used the broken glass to make glass beads with a local artist; I've saved the lids to make sun catchers, but at the moment, I use them to weight must bags in home wine making.
4. This emptied commercial marmalade jar once held homemade marmalade, then served as our first yeast expander; currently, it holds our collection of beach glass.
5. Glass gallon jar and lid. The jar currently holds bulk sweetener. The lid in the drainer has been drilled for a stopper and airlock, to make a primary fermenter for home wine making.

In addition, you can see a plastic container and lid that have been reused many times for a variety of tasks.

The only really limiting factor in glass containers is the lid. Metal and plastic have less longevity than glass.

Even so, there are other ways to secure a glass container that is missing its original lid. It just takes a little forethought and ingenuity.

Glass is a lot sturdier than we're taught to believe. What action movie would be complete without a bottle broken over someone's head, or someone getting thrown through a plate glass window? In the real world, most people hit over the head with a bottle go down hard with a serious injury, while the bottle doesn't even chip. Most of the glass containers in your home will outlive you.

Glass can and does break, of course. When we break a glass container, we put it in the recycling bin, but rarely before.

Originally posted on The Zeiger Family Homestead Blog March 21, 2012.

Repurposing Old Wall Calendars

On New Year's Day, I spent a few minutes performing what has become an annual chore: cutting up the previous year's wall calendar to save the art for future projects.

I take an inordinate amount of time to seek out an acceptable calendar to see me through each year. I really enjoy having a pleasant calendar on my wall, in a calendar frame. It's art that changes every month. I choose them with care, making sure the one I select is worth having for a whole year. In fact, when the year has passed, I'm reluctant to give the artwork up.

Which is why I often don't.

I've come too late to reusing calendar art. I've thrown away a lot of good calendars over the years; some I'd really like to have back, but never will.

I admit, I don't recycle calendars, which is the most obvious way to reuse a good calendar. There are a finite number of day and date combinations. These can cycle around again in as little as six years, short enough to make it worth storing a calendar, long enough that the artwork will seem fresh and new again. All one has to do is make sure one doesn't forget what year it is. If one can't, it's easy to write the current year over the old one!

I generally have other plans for the calendar. I like to cut them up and use them for projects. I definitely save the main artwork, but often use the covers, edges and trimmings as well.

I'm building a couple of frames that will allow me to display one or two seasonally appropriate pictures throughout the year. I've made greeting cards, wrapping paper, and stuck artwork into the fronts of binders. Once I cut out the "thumbnails" of several years' artwork and lined them up by month. I use these to mark a book of days I consult daily throughout each year, switching to a new bookmark each month.

None of this solves any urgent problems; and, even with the cost of some printed calendars, I'm not being extremely frugal by repurposing a calendar after its year comes and goes. But, I find satisfaction in the crafts I make with them, and I love keeping around the artwork I chose so carefully in the past to enjoy in the future.

Originally posted on The Zeiger Family Homestead Blog January 2, 2013.

Eating Alaska: **A documentary Explores "Eating Locally" in a Locale Not So Near You**

Late last January we hiked to town to see *Eating Alaska*, a documentary by Ellen Frankenstein (no, really!) about eating locally.

Ellen, who lives in Sitka, explores what it means to feed one's self and one's family in Alaska, where our food supply is a strange mixture. On the one hand we have commercially available foods like everyone else, most of which arrive on a (fairly) reliable basis from elsewhere, often from the other side of the world.

On the other hand, we have our indigenous foods, a cornucopia of plants and animals free for the taking, although that taking requires a great deal of effort from us. The majority of Alaskans can make a choice between the two.

Most opt for commercially available foods, while others, like many in the Native villages, and non-Natives like Ellen and her partner, choose to procure their own food as much as possible. This struck a chord with my family, as we're trying to do the same.

The film is very informative as well as entertaining. Ellen's ambivalence about hunting, her contemplation of the questions raised by taking lives to sustain one's own, the challenges of gardening in rainy Southeast Alaska are all handled with understated humor and charm, supported by whimsical captioning and graphics. Ellen travels around Alaska, talking to farmers in the MatSu Valley, home of Alaska's legendary giant vegetables, visiting with Native students in Kotzebue High School's home-ec class, attending a "culture camp," and hunting and fishing in various regions.

Her interviews revealed a generally healthy attitude toward food among Alaskans. Particularly encouraging, and somewhat unexpected in this modern age, is one young man's comment that he prefers to eat hunted meat because he wants to know who processed his food. That's an attitude few of his fellow Americans take, preferring that their meat come to them cleanly and neatly packaged without any hints as to what steps were taken to bring it to their table.

Frankenstein visits with a group of vegetarians who discuss their "oddball" status in a population that eats so much wild game and fish. Other highlights include Ellen's rallying effort to "talk down" her panicking camera operator when the scheduled pickup flight from a remote hunt fails to show up for a few days, and an interview with a wickedly deadpan Tlingit elder.

Particularly pleasing to me, I discovered that Ellen is friends with a friend of mine from junior high and high school. This young woman helps Ellen try to come to terms with hunting, taking her to hunt deer, caribou and mountain goat, and helping her get used to hunting equipment.

Even if you don't know anyone in the film, watching *Eating Alaska* will teach you a lot about what it means to eat locally, and get a flavor (if you will) for life in Alaska.

The film's scenes of Alaskan wildlife and geography are wonderful. The faint-at-heart should be warned: the film contains scenes of processing meat, seafood and, yes, vegetables. There are some fairly straightforward hunting scenes, including an "unclean kill." These scenes are integral to the film's considerations, and are an important aspect of the narrative. Nothing is dwelt on, it's just presented for what it is: a part of life and death. If you're unwilling to accept that, don't worry—the camera "turns away" from most of the actual killing.

You can get information on the film at Ellen's Web site, www.EatingAlaska.com. This would be an excellent presentation for gardening and hunting clubs, or any group discussing eating locally, if only because it shows how we do it in Alaska.

Originally posted on The Zeiger Family Homestead Blog October 7, 2009.

Bath from the Past: Using an Ewer and Basin

Our family first learned how easy and pleasant it is to use an ewer and basin long before we moved to the homestead. We tried it while visiting friends who served as winter caretakers for a summer camp near Juneau. They spent most of the day without power, firing up the camp's generators for only an hour or two each day. No power meant no pumps, so they used an ewer and basin for personal washing most of the time, and we learned to do likewise.

Despite what one used to modern convenience might assume, "sponge bathing," as my parents called it, is not a bad way to wash. The thick porcelain or crockery of the ewer and basin holds heat surprisingly well, allowing ample time for a thorough, even leisurely wash without the water getting cold. Further, even I, who at the time depended on gallons of water for an "adequate" shower, found a pitcher full of water more than enough for my needs with very little strategic planning or frugal usage.

We liked it. As a gift for Michelle, Aly and I went to a local ceramics shop, chose, cleaned up, glazed, and fired an ewer and basin set. Of all Aly's and my various projects, this one might be the most fun so far. We worked together on it, and Aly, who was 5 at the time, made a doll-sized set for herself, which she decorated with hand painted flowers. Even if the set never proved useful, I'll always cherish those hours.

Now that we've moved to the homestead, even though we can make hot water for showers with our wood-fired water heater, we don't always choose to do so;

instead, we heat water on the stove and fill the ewer. Or, we may use hot water from a thermos that's cooled too much for hot drinks, but is still warm enough for washing. The ewer and basin can easily be carried to any room for greater privacy or convenience.

We've acquired another set for the guesthouse (they're a common thrift shop or garage sale item). We're always on the look out for more, just in case.

Once again, we've discovered through use how practical an "outmoded" technology can be.

Originally posted on The Zeiger Family Homestead Blog July 21, 2010.

The Giving Tree

The local variety of birch is our most precious wood resource on the "homestead." While its harvest can be highly problematic, it's well worth the effort. A birch, in many ways, is similar to Shel Silverstein's *Giving Tree*.

Consider:

I was surprised to find that the most recent birch I felled is hollow through much of its length. While this means we'll miss out on some of the volume of solid firewood, there are other advantages.

The rotten wood that fills the hollow spaces is rich, natural compost. I excavated the stump with an army surplus trenching tool, and scooped the insides of the hollow branches clean. Roughly speaking, I filled three 5-gallon buckets with wood duff. All of it can go right on the garden beds, a real boon for us, gardening on thin soil as we do.

The firewood produced from the tree is still considerable. I got several solid rounds from the main trunk. The sound upper branches yielded rounds of good stove wood; the highest branches, already bone dry, will serve nicely as kindling. The twigs, chips from felling, miscellaneous small fragments and the outer wood of the stump yield buckets of fuel for our hot water heater. The bark is excellent for fires; the thin, papery parts are better than newspaper for tinder, the thick slabs from the base of the tree burn well and long. Any bark that stays on the logs will help them ignite in a fire, what falls off can be gathered for tinder.

The bucking, gathering, hauling, chopping, and stacking all provide vital exercise outside in the fresh air.

The tree's fragrance is heavenly. It clings to my hands, arms, and clothing at the end of the day, and perfumes the forest around me. The sweet smoke that will rise when we burn it this coming winter will be like incense.

Through all of this processing, I've been careful to avoid damaging the lone sucker that has sprouted from the underground section of the old tree's roots. Green, slender, and reaching for the sunlight, with luck, it'll grow until, some 15 to 20 years from now, it will become a giving tree for Aly and her children.

Originally posted on The Zeiger Family Homestead Blog April 23, 2012.

The Paradigm's Pay-Off

If I've managed to include all the posts from our blog that best outline or explain our paradigm, strategies and mind set, then most of the remaining posts could be included here to show how we benefit from choosing this lifestyle. Rather than do that, I've chosen a few key posts that convey some of the joy this life brings us.

Killer Whales in Lynn Canal

Sunday afternoon we watched a flock of Barrow's goldeneyes, a type of sea duck, fish off our rocks. The current tide cycle's highs are around 20 feet, so they congregated right at the rocky edge where we could see them well. As they moved south, the windbreak obscured them slightly.

We heard a rushing sound that confused us for a moment. It sounded like a humpback whale blow, but it was truncated. We then decided that what we'd heard was the rush of the ducks' wings—something had spooked them. Then, a black sickle cut the water out in the canal.

Killer whales!

We grabbed coats and binoculars, and scrambled out the door down to the beach. A pod of killer whales swept past, dispersed widely across the canal, some near the far shore, two miles or more away, some mid-fjord. Suddenly, a group of three—two juveniles and a massive male, with a dorsal fin rising some six feet above the water—surfaced and blew within 100 yards of where we stood.

Neighbors once told us that we should keep an eye out for killer whales toward the end of January and beginning of February. They said a certain pod seemed to have a habit of coming up Lynn Canal about then. Every year since, we've seen them come by. They come at other times too, and it's always a special treat, a spectacle.

We counted somewhere around ten individuals of all ages and both sexes (killer whale females have shorter, sickle-shaped dorsal fins, mature males have the impossibly tall dorsal). They moved fast, apparently traveling rather than feeding. We're never sure whether we're seeing the fish-eating "residents" or mammal eating "transients" unless we actually see them hunting. Both types of killer whales frequent the area, although we've only confirmed residents from our homestead, as they feed on herring runs.

Seeing killer whales is always exhilarating. We never get tired of watching them, especially the mature bulls. That tall dorsal pops out of the water for long seconds before the head appears, then lingers long on the dive. We've never seen the droopy dorsal of captive or sick orcas here.

That evening, they passed on their way back south in the dark. With no wind, the sound of their exhalations filled the air—we couldn't see them, or tell from the sound how close or how far away they were. We heard the noise from inside the cabin. Outside, it sounded like they were about to jump into our laps. We'd hoped they might stay up north a bit, then pass us during the day, so we could see them again. We'll just have to be patient, and wait for next time.

Originally posted on The Zeiger Family Homestead Blog February 3, 2010.

Everything is Illuminated

The title of a movie I like came repeatedly to mind during a recent stretch of sunny weather: *Everything Is Illuminated.*

Indeed, it was.

Bright sunshine flooding our forest, combined with the seasonally rapid increase in the amount of daylight each day, cast a glow over our landscape that became positively disorienting. Repeatedly, during the period, I became "lost" in the forest, unable to recognize my surroundings, even as I followed known landmarks on a well-used trail.

Quality of light has a major impact on our view. Subtle shifts in light can change a vista in significant ways. Close at hand, this leads to rather comical conversations on the trail, as one or the other of us asks such inane questions as: "Has this rock always been here?"

The familiar becomes alien in slightly different light. We often find ourselves lingering along the trail to stare about us, watching as new features become highlighted, while others fade into the background.

This is why we have so many photos of The Mountain with No Name across the fjord. It changes dramatically as the day's light moves across it.

Following a neighbor's trail home from the bay, I thought about this as I alternated between admiring the sunlit forest and staring at it distrustfully. I considered taking a photograph to accompany a blog post much like this one, but then I realized it would have no significance for anyone who isn't here, who doesn't use these trails as we do. Such a one would have no sense of the change that I see as I make my way through the comfortably familiar, made slightly uncomfortable by a different light.

Originally posted on The Zeiger Family Homestead Blog May 19, 2011.

A Good Haul

The life of the homestead must continue on all fronts. Progress is uneven, but continual. Yesterday, thanks to some extra effort, we are reaping significant benefits.

I went to town with Michelle to run some errands when she went to work on Wednesday.

On Tuesday afternoon's high tide, I had launched the canoe from the homestead and paddled around to where our kayak sits on the shore of Mud Bay. I hopped in the kayak and towed the canoe to the roadside, where I beached it and returned across the bay by kayak. This put the canoe in position to receive cargo Wednesday evening.

We had two empty propane tanks ready for refilling. We saw an opportunity to haul all that weight by sea.

We also expected that a periodic bulk order through Michelle's work would arrive that day, so we knew we'd likely have a full canoe, and a good high tide for hauling. We also anticipated more of the same calm, windless weather we've experienced the past few weeks. Michelle's last appointment of the day would end at full slack tide. I would rendezvous with her with filled tanks and other goods in time to catch it.

This plan began to seem doubtful when we heard the day's marine forecast: 25-knot winds by evening. We've learned that if and when winds develop, they reach our peninsula earlier than the broadcast predicts. We would have to watch to see if we still had calm waters, and travel with a weather eye open, as always, ready to ditch at one of several possible landings around the point should the wind become too strong.

A breeze had definitely developed in Mud Bay by the time we arrived and loaded the canoe. Wind tends to funnel through there at greater intensity than the surrounding waters, so we decided to launch, expecting less wind out in the fjord, but planning to ditch if necessary.

Paddling against the wind with a full load isn't easy, but we had no real difficulty. We faced an increasing chop, requiring us to paddle fast enough to plow over or through waves before they slopped into the boat. The worst conditions came at the mouth of the bay, where the first of the out flowing tide met the opposing wind, and made the water boil around us.

Then came the crucial stretch: skirting the point itself. The most direct route would require us to allow the swell and chop to hit us broadside, which is unwise. Instead, I steered a course out into Lynn Canal, diagonal to the point of land and the oncoming chop. It also forced us to face into the rising wind.

As Michelle threw all her effort into paddling, I ticked off the safe beaching points as they passed, trying to calculate if and when to run for shore and safety.

We knew that after we doubled the last small tip of the point, we could turn sharply and ride the south wind home, paddling more easily, only making sure that we didn't get "pooped" by the following sea.

When I called out for Michelle to paddle hard as I swung the bow around, she felt the great relief of knowing the hard part was over. I had seen something that made me realize that may not be so.

A large cruise ship powered south through Lynn Canal ahead of us. We would intersect its wake sometime before we reached home.

Most of these massive ships are designed to minimize wake. We've seen bigger wakes generated by the far smaller Alaska Marine Highway ferries than from some of the big tour ships. However, a lot of factors come into play in determining the size of wake each ship generates. Usually, they pass our property fairly slowly, but some power on through, and the resulting waves can be massive as they hit our shore. And, many times, the wakes are strong enough to crest out in the fjord, despite the deep water.

I could see a few local fishing boats dotting the water ahead of us. The tour ship's heading angled somewhat from west to east as it came south, indicating that the ship would avoid the fishing ground, and probably travel a bit slower to keep from rattling the fisherfolk too much. These signs gave us hope.

We consulted briefly, shouting above the noise of wind and waves. We could make for the last good beach on the coast and "ditch," landing our canoe and its load ahead of the ship's wake.

This would be difficult for a variety of reasons. The wake would gain energy as the sloping beach tripped up the waveform, crashing down as surf on the beach and anything on it.

If we ditched, we would need to drag the fully loaded canoe far enough up the cobble beach to clear the surging waves. We would then have to prioritize the load. We could leave the cargo in the canoe, provided we pulled it above the next high tide line. We'd need to tarp it against the weather, and haul overland anything that might attract bears or other critters.

Better to stand off the shore and ride out the wake before putting in to our homestead beach. In the deep water, the wake would most likely be a large, smooth swell—unless it curled and broke.

We decided to risk it, and continued up the coast, slacking our pace a bit. We were eager to arrive, but knew we couldn't land until after the wake passed.

By then, the wind had increased to a fairly steady 20 knots (23 m.p.h.), and the swell had grown to the point that even a tour ship wake seemed somewhat academic.

However, with the wind and sea at our back, we bobbed along in relative peace, keeping a sharp eye out for the approaching wake.

When it came, we were gratified to find it a large but smooth rollercoaster ride that lasted a few minutes, then passed. Watching it sweep the shoreline, we could see that, as tour ship wakes go, this one was fairly gentle. We gave it time to settle, then landed below our boat deck.

As we touched shore, Michelle leapt from the bow with our long painter in hand. Watching the waves behind me for my chance, I scrambled over the load and the bow, removing my weight from the stern before a wave could "poop" us.

We hustled our cargo up to the covered porch of the boathouse, dragged the canoe to the deck, flipped it, and tied its painter.

Throughout the adventure, rain fell steadily. We managed to keep our cargo dry for the most part, but we were soaked to the skin. Once we secured our gear, we rushed to the cabin, traded wet clothes for dry, fuzzy bathrobes, and started dinner.

We had weathered an intense stretch of activity in less than optimal conditions, but we liked the pay off: a good supply of food and other supplies, two full propane tanks, and a new set of three cast iron skillets in graduated sizes, a treasure found at our local second hand store. At the end of it all, we found ourselves safe and sound in the heart of the homestead.

It doesn't get much better than this.

Originally posted on The Zeiger Family Homestead Blog August 23 and 24, 2012.

Skies on Fire

Every once in a while, insomnia can be a good thing. I had to get up early in the night for a "relief break," rising just after midnight. I almost always get up in the night—an easy indicator that I'm drinking enough liquids during the day—but I usually get up between 2:30 and 4:30 a.m.

I stepped out under a brilliant, starlit sky. Without urban light pollution, we easily see the Milky Way over our homestead.

I went out to the veranda to look north. I saw aurora borealis, a hazy glowing band along the tops of the mountains. Nice, but not worth sticking around for, so I went back to bed.

About two hours later, Michelle woke me to see the northern lights. By then, the display had developed to the point that it was definitely worth getting up to see.

The northern half of the sky, from the horizon somewhere over Skagway, to the sky above LC Mountain, appeared to be on fire. Shafts and curtains of light developed and disappeared in rapid succession. At times it appeared as giant, pale green candle flames. Higher above our heads, the arcs seemed to follow the patterns shown in depictions of Earth's magnetic field.

The vast display could not be taken in all at once. We had to turn and look all around us to try to see everything. While we focused on one area of movement, another, more dramatic sight developed elsewhere. We settled down on our "veranda" seat, tilted our heads back, and snuggled, enjoying the show.

Michelle hadn't been able to sleep since I'd returned to bed earlier. A restless cat and thoughts of the approaching workday had kept sleep away. A session in the cool, fresh air, enjoying a fantastic display of northern lights, did the trick. When we returned to bed, she slept soundly till well past sunrise.

The University of Alaska Geophysical Institute's Aurora Forecast listed last night's activity as "low." Tonight's forecast is for "medium." I think I'll go pour another glass of water....

Originally posted on The Zeiger Family Homestead Blog March 27, 2012.

A Bad Day Fishing

You know the saying, "a bad day fishing beats a good day at the office." I've tested the limits of that old saw lately.

Conditions aren't optimal at the moment. The tides are at the low end of the cycle. The mid-morning high barely reaches my favorite ledge, so landing a catch is harder and less sure.

The horse and deer flies are relentless, biting through my clothes and adding a rather spastic play to my lure as I try to retrieve it while laying about me in a frantic effort to kill flies.

The bladder wrack seaweed is on the move, drifting in rafts with the current and snagging on virtually every cast.

And, oddly, the large Dolly Varden char seem to have disappeared, so that the fingerlings are the only ones around to bite the lure. Their enthusiastic feeding, jumping out of the water all around me, just adds false excitement to the process, heaping insult on injury.

I've lost three of my favorite, most expensive lures in the last two days.

Over it all, the relentless sunshine burns me as I spend hours trying to catch a single fish.

I'm not a particularly superstitious person, but I do believe in irony. I felt a twinge of apprehension when I blogged previously that we were almost guaranteed a fish for any meal I fished for. The evidence seems clear: I jinxed myself!

And yet, I can't stop trying. I love the rhythm of shore casting, and even the remotest possibility of catching a fish is too enticing to ignore.

Besides, the pay-off is excellent. With health experts saying we should all eat more fish, what could be more worthwhile than making the effort to catch a healthy, fresh-as-can-be meal for free? Win or lose, the end justifies the sometimes-frustrating means.

Besides, it can't last. The weather will turn wet, improving fishing conditions; the Dollies will return. Soon the salmon will begin moving through in greater numbers. It's a dry spell, but my luck will change soon. I've just got to keep trying.

Any time I get too discouraged, I compare this work to the kind I used to do, in an office.

The old saying is right on the money!

Originally posted on The Zeiger Family Homestead Blog June 11, 2010.

"Lost Lake" Ramble

Yesterday, for Aly's birthday, she and I indulged in one of our favorite activities: rambling.

We had the day to ourselves, as Michelle filled in for a coworker on her part-time job, so we threw a lunch, some water, and a canister of bear spray in a daypack, and headed up the ridge along the "moose highway".

In 2009, a friend and I hiked up there scouting for moose before the season opened. We saw two things on that hike that Aly and I have been searching for, off and on, ever since: a small lake or large pond (which my friend had seen before) and a really nice little cave (which my friend had not seen before). We've never been able to find either again, including yesterday, but we have a lot of fun trying.

We hiked up the ridge for a couple of hours, following a trail that a neighbor had improved recently, chainsawing windfalls off the path, and refreshing some of the blazes.

We followed blazes till they ran out, then started casting back and forth across the ridge, looking for the lake. We found some spectacular overlooks of the Katzehin delta across Lynn Canal, and got close enough to the road on the other side of the ridge that we could hear it, if not see it.

We made our own way home rather than trying to relocate the trail. That led us to some interesting places, remembered and half-remembered from previous rambles. We found a gully that I had seen before, that appears almost to be hewn purposely out of the rock. We also found a knoll where we'd once shared a picnic lunch.

As we gazed down the length of our peninsula, recognizing landmarks, we despaired of getting home by 4:00 pm, as we'd told Michelle we would.

Nevertheless, we set off through the woods, navigating mostly by intuition. Before long we found the trail again, and made our way home.

We're not sure exactly how long it took—Aly said I had told her we had 15 minutes to our deadline, but I really doubt we could have gone that far in such short time, with no trail most of the way.

At any rate, we arrived home on time, and had preparations for Aly's birthday dinner started when Michelle stepped through the door 5 minutes later.

Eventually, we'll find the lake, but I'm beginning to wonder if we'll ever find the cave.

I'm also beginning to wonder if we really want to?

Originally posted on The Zeiger Family Homestead Blog July 23, 2011.

Coffee With a Whale

Yesterday morning, I sat at the edge of our rocks. Cat's paws rippled the water's still surface; pale spring sunshine bathed the mountains and me, while wisps of cloud shrouded their peaks.

On the "Power Point" behind me, our solar array glinted. The blades of the wind generator turned with majestic slowness as its bullet nose swung back and forth, as if sniffing out a breeze.

I sipped coffee from my favorite mug. Sea lions at Gran Point, a few miles across Lynn Canal, growled and howled, as ever. Three ruby crowned kinglets interrupted each other's songs in the trees behind me. Somewhere in the Coast Range an avalanche banged its way into a ravine.

Greatly magnified, the mostly unnamed mountains seemed to swell until they hung above me, threatening to fall. The morning's freshness, salt tang and warming spruce and hemlock, with a touch of birch and alder bud, sweetened my morning "mug up."

Every so often, spaced just enough to make me start slightly with its sudden appearance and deep "whoosh" of breath, a humpback whale surfaced beneath me, slowly, almost lazily working its way through our bight in large loops.

The herring run has started!

We've been expecting it, but "the Next Big Thing" took us a bit by surprise on Thursday. Since the herring fishery closed in Sitka, we'd been watching for signs of approaching shoals: gathering whales, excited sea lions, and clouds of sea birds. Usually, all of these appear in increasing numbers, and excitement builds until, at last, the herring begin to gather and spawn.

This year, things happened a bit differently. We'd seen a whale or two, recently. Sea lions had only just begun to swim in larger, noisier groups. I began to think about overhauling the nets. I'd guessed we had another week at least, perhaps more, before the herring arrived.

The night of the 14th, and again the next morning, we heard whales. Around 10:30 a pair of them swam north, where a large pod of harbor porpoises joined them. The whales began feeding, and the porpoises raced through the water around them. As we watched at the water's edge, a small shoal of herring swam past our feet.

Aly and I scrambled. We didn't run for the nets; the shoal was too small. Instead, she grabbed her hydrophone and recording gear. I'd been thinking about how to improve its performance, and tried several ideas. As a reward, we listened to the herring (which make a clicking sound, like a Geiger counter) and the two whales as they passed close by. They apparently don't vocalize much while feeding, although if we're lucky, they might bubble net later on. We heard slight sounds and the rush of water as they passed. Excitement enough for now!

Our urgency to catch herring will increase soon. Until then, yesterday brought plenty of other jobs to tend to, and soon I had to break my reverie and move on. But to sit for a while and enjoy my morning coffee in the company of a whale was heavenly!

Originally posted on The Zeiger Family Homestead Blog April 17, 2010. Reprinted in New Homesteading Magazine, Issue #1 April 2011.

EPILOGUE: THE ADVENTURE CONTINUES

It's hard to say, at this point in our lives, where our adventure will lead us next. Aly is in college, beginning to explore the possibilities of adult life. Even though she currently plans to return to the "homestead" to build a place of her own—perhaps a tree house—we are considering our next steps with the possibility that our family team will be reduced to two. We have many different plans to improve the homestead, from rearranging living arrangements in the cabin to constructing additional outbuildings. We may get around to trying to raise chickens. We'll continue to develop micro incomes, including items to sell on our Website store and more books about our life—maybe even a cookbook? We will eventually realize many of these plans; others will never come to fruition. Despite days when I just don't want to do it anymore, no doubt the blog will continue. As new developments arise, one may read about them there.

If you've been inspired by our example, create your own plan. Take the first steps toward living the life you would live, no matter what that might be. There's no sense waiting until conditions are perfect; they never will be. It's up to each of us to make the conditions favorable enough for us to work toward, and achieve our goals. It won't be easy, but it will be satisfying!

About the Author

Mark A. Zeiger has lived in Alaska, his native state, for most of his life. He now lives a mostly subsistence lifestyle on his semi-remote, off-the-grid "homestead" on the shore of Lynn Canal, south of Haines. He designs Websites and blogs about his family's homestead life at AKZeigers.com. He has previously released a collection of dark fiction short stories, *Shy Ghosts Dancing: Dark Tales from Southeast Alaska*. He lives with his wife, Michelle, their daughter, Aly, and their cat, Spice.

Look for more books about the Zeiger Family Homestead in the future. You'll find them and more at the Zeiger Family Homestead Website Store: AKZeigers.com/store.html.

* * * *

The electricity used to write, edit, and design *Sacred Coffee: A "Homesteader's" Paradigm* came exclusively from alternative sources—wind and solar power generated on the Zeiger's off-the-grid "homestead."

Made in the USA
Middletown, DE
02 June 2023

31923926R00099